SUICIDE

SUICIDE

UNDERSTANDING AND ENDING
A NATIONAL TRAGEDY

JOHN BATESON

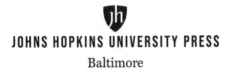

JOHNS HOPKINS UNIVERSITY PRESS

Baltimore

© 2024 Johns Hopkins University Press
All rights reserved. Published 2024
Printed in the United States of America on acid-free paper
9 8 7 6 5 4 3 2 1

Johns Hopkins University Press
2715 North Charles Street
Baltimore, Maryland 21218
www.press.jhu.edu

Library of Congress Cataloging-in-Publication Data is available.

A catalog record for this book is available from the British Library.

ISBN 978-1-4214-4941-8 (hardcover)
ISBN 978-1-4214-4943-2 (ebook)

Special discounts are available for bulk purchases of this book. For more information, please contact Special Sales at specialsales@jh.edu.

Actually, it was only part of myself I wanted to kill—the part that wanted to kill herself, that dragged me into the suicide debate and made every window, kitchen implement, and subway station a rehearsal for tragedy.

—SUSANNA KAYSEN, *GIRL, INTERRUPTED*

A phenomenon that a number of people have noted while in deep depression is the sense of being accompanied by a second self—a wraithlike observer who, not sharing the dementia of his double, is able to watch with dispassionate curiosity as his companion struggles against the oncoming disaster, or decides to embrace it. There is a theatrical quality about all this, and during the next several days, as I went about stolidly preparing for extinction, I couldn't shake off a sense of melodrama—a melodrama in which I, the victim to be of self-murder, was both the solitary actor and lone member of the audience.

—WILLIAM STYRON, *DARKNESS INVISIBLE*

Contents

SUICIDE

Introduction

FEW SUBJECTS ARE AS MISUNDERSTOOD AS SUICIDE. For family members, the stigma of suicide causes feelings of shame and embarrassment that rarely accompany other types of death. Anger, guilt, and confusion enter into it as well, leading people to hush up a suicide or refer to it as an accident or the result of an undefined, health-related condition. Even when someone's suicide is known by many, it rarely is acknowledged as such in obituaries. Instead, the person "died suddenly," and there is no reference to the manner of death.

In most parts of the world, including the United States, suicide is considered to be a mental health problem. People who are suicidal are treated through psychotherapy and medications. The therapy helps individuals see the harmful effects of their behavior and how to change it, while the medications offset chemical imbalances that result in depression, mood swings, and other psychological disorders. At least that is the theory. In practice, the success of therapy depends on how open the individual is to it and how skilled the therapist is in providing it, while the effectiveness of pills rests on the accuracy of the diagnosis and the relevance of the prescription.

Thinking of suicide solely in terms of mental health narrows the focus to the level of the individual. If one views suicide through a broader lens, however, it's not only appropriate but necessary to consider it a public health problem with large-scale social consequences. That is where my focus, and the focus of this book, lies.

To understand suicide—and more importantly, to end it—we must adopt a far-reaching point of view. We must look at the impact of stigma and how it discourages many suicidal people from seeking help. We must look at steps that society can take to reduce easy access to lethal means. We must ensure that health care professionals are trained to identify people at risk of suicide and to intervene effectively.

For a person who has never seriously contemplated suicide, it's hard to imagine what that is like. It's possible with the aid of props to grasp the consequences of aging when one is still young. Special glasses that approximate cataracts, earplugs that block out most sounds, and knee braces that limit mobility provide a sense of what many elderly people deal with on a daily basis. There aren't any props, however, that enable a fully functioning person to experience mental illness. We aren't able to get inside the mind of someone who is living with clinically diagnosed depression. Most of us do have experience in dealing with the breakup of a relationship, the death of a loved one, financial troubles, legal issues, a drinking problem, or drug abuse—all triggers for suicide. Even so, in most instances such experiences don't lead to a prolonged sense of hopelessness that things are never going to get better. Our emotional pain isn't so great that it overrides everything else, seemingly forever. For some people, though, it does, to the point where relief is the only thing that matters.

The vast majority of people who kill themselves don't want to die. Rather, they want an end to their pain, be it mental, physical, or emotional, and they believe that suicide is the only way this will happen. Usually there are other options, but they aren't able to see them because their thinking is impaired. It's up to the rest of us—as individuals and as a society—to help.

A good way to start is by examining the terminology we use when talking about suicide. It's common for people to say that someone *committed suicide*. This implies that killing yourself is illegal, however, when it's not. People commit crimes like robbery or rape or murder, but there is no law against suicide. Referring to suicide in this way adds to the stigma; it implies that the person did something wrong. Instead, we need to take judgment out of it. We need to stop thinking of suicide as wrong and accept it for what it is: an individual's decision to end his or her life prematurely. We don't say that someone *committed cancer*, even when his or her actions—such as cigarette smoking for years—may have had a direct effect. Instead we say that the person *died by cancer*, and this is the way we should refer to suicide: the person *died by suicide*. Alternatively, it's appropriate to say that someone killed himself or herself. No judgment; just fact.

"It comes back to how we can speak of our dead with love and compassion," says the mother of a 21-year-old boy who took his own life. "Saying that your loved one *committed suicide* seems like the ultimate act of betrayal—blaming them for their own illness and suffering. Bring them back to the light, your conversation, your family history, your mantel or photo album, with loving compassion by proclaiming that they died *by suicide*. . . . They were ill, they ended their pain, and we mourn them."[1]

It's also inappropriate to say that a person who attempts suicide either *succeeds*—that is, dies—or *fails*—lives. Again, we need to avoid judging. Moreover, suicide shouldn't be thought of as a goal, like passing or failing a test. An individual survives a suicide attempt or doesn't. If the latter, it's referred to as a *completed suicide*.

My Story

Until 1996, when I was hired as executive director of a nationally certified crisis-intervention and suicide-prevention center in the San Francisco Bay Area, I knew relatively little about suicide. Up to that time my primary source of information had been Émile Durkheim's book *Suicide*, published a hundred years earlier and required reading in university sociology classes. No one in my immediate family nor any close friends had killed themselves. Despite growing up only a few minutes away from the world's number-one suicide site—the Golden Gate Bridge—it was easy for me to go about my daily life with little thought of people who were contemplating death.

My background was in social services, and I applied for the job because I thought it would be enlightening, challenging, and personally satisfying—which it was. What I lacked in knowledge about the agency's work I made up for in skills and experience in other areas, and I believed that I would learn what I needed to know fairly quickly.

A few months after I started, I completed the agency's hotline training program and began answering crisis calls. After a time, I was elected to the steering committee of the National Suicide Prevention Lifeline (now known as the 988 Suicide and Crisis Lifeline). I also was appointed to a blue-ribbon committee that created the *California Strategic Plan on Suicide Prevention*. Later, I was a presenter at annual conferences of the American Association of Suicidology and the National Association of Crisis Center Directors.

When I left the crisis center after sixteen years, I received a special commendation from the California legislature. I also wrote a book, *Building Hope*, in which I recounted some of my experiences. More importantly, I began implementing plans to turn what I had learned into tools for change. First up was to increase public awareness of suicides from the Golden Gate Bridge.

My book *The Final Leap* was the first book written about Golden Gate Bridge suicides. Of the dozens of books written about the bridge, a few had mentioned bridge suicides, but none had focused on the problem. In the aftermath of the book's publication, money was raised and work began on a physical deterrent to future bridge suicides, a marine-grade, stainless steel net. The advocacy of family members who had lost loved ones to the bridge had more impact than anything else on getting the net approved and funded, but my book played a part, mainly by telling their stories.

It was followed by *The Last and Greatest Battle*. It too was a first: the first book devoted exclusively to the problem of military suicides. The impetus for the book was the increasing number of suicides by active-duty service members and veterans. By 2014, on average one US soldier, sailor, airman, or Marine died by suicide every day.[2] The number of veterans' suicides is even more alarming, with one veteran dying by suicide nearly every hour.[3] Veterans constitute 10 percent of the US population, but they account for more than 20 percent of all suicides in the country.[4] According to a study in 2021 by the Cost of War Project, since 9/11 four times as many service members have died by suicide as have died in combat.[5]

As the problem worsened and the number of calls from suicidal veterans and family members to agencies like mine skyrocketed, I wanted to learn more about it, but I couldn't find a book devoted to the subject. There were many books about war but few that mentioned suicide. Moreover, the ones that did mention it offered little analysis and few recommendations for dealing with the problem effectively.

I never served in the military, but I did know something about suicide by this time, and I approached the problem from that perspective. Also, I thought that what I had to say was important and was not being said by anyone else. It remains to be seen whether any of my recommendations are adopted, but at least they are generating conversations.

My most recent book, *The Education of a Coroner*, focused on the work of coroners in general and one coroner in particular. A coroner's work is different from what is depicted on most TV shows, and few people know anything about it until the day comes when a coroner knocks on their door and delivers news that will change their lives forever.

Coroners often start out having little regard for people who kill themselves. Coroners have so many other deaths to deal with—deaths of individuals who didn't want to die—that it's hard for them to have much compassion for people who take their own lives. After years of meeting with the families of suicide victims, however, and reading the poignant notes that have been left behind, notes explaining the person's troubles and formidable barriers to a healthy life, many coroners form a different opinion. They realize that there are major holes in our health care system today.

This Book

The present book, unlike other books on suicide, is not targeted at clinicians or medical professionals who treat suicidal individuals. It's also not targeted at grief counselors who try to console people after the suicide of a loved one. Some of the information may benefit people in these fields, but the intended audience is broader and less knowledgeable about suicide.

This book also differs from others in that it's not a first-person account of a suicidal mind. I don't attempt to shed light on the problem of suicide through a personal story of darkness and despair. The books that do this have much to offer in the way of insight and understanding, and they communicate important lessons that someone has learned. They rarely advocate for meaningful solutions to the problem of suicide, however, which is where my interest lies.

The more we learn about suicide, the less taboo it becomes and the more our misperceptions disappear. Penny Coleman, the widow of a Vietnam veteran who killed himself, calls suicide "the secret death" because people don't want to talk about it, yet everyone has an opinion. Attitudes have fluctuated, she says, regarding whether suicide is "a sin, a right, a crime, a romantic gesture, an act of consummate bravery, or a symptom of mental illness. It has never, however, been an emotionally neutral issue."[6]

Changing attitudes is the first step in ending suicides, but only the first step. To arrive at policy changes and cultural shifts, a number of interim steps are required, starting with education and public awareness. Because so much misinformation about suicide exists, it's important to make the truth known. That is why the chapter "Fiction vs. Fact" leads off this book. It's followed by "The Proverbial Question," dealing with the question asked by everyone after someone they know dies by suicide, *Why?* Demographics of suicide—who, where, when, and how, including the effect of COVID-19 on suicide—are presented in chapter 3, "By the Numbers," with a particular emphasis on youths, seniors, Native Americans, and the LGBTQ community. Chapter 4, "Special Situations," covers suicide in unique settings—parks, prisons, the military—as well as assisted suicide, suicide by cop, and murder-suicide, which includes mass shootings. Chapter 5, "Talking to a Suicidal Person," concludes the first half of the book and is a guide to what may be the single most meaningful conversation anyone has with someone who is contemplating suicide.

In the second half of the book the focus shifts to an essential element in suicide prevention, restricting access to lethal means. Specifically, it describes the relationship between guns and suicide, drugs and suicide, and jump sites and suicide. Knowing the role that firearms, pills, and unrestricted high places play in suicide attempts is critical to preventing people from killing themselves. Guns are the most common method of suicide in this country, accounting for more than half of all suicide deaths. Drugs aren't quite as lethal, but 70 percent of all suicide attempts are the result of pills and other drugs. Jumps are farther down the list, both in terms of attempts and in terms of the number of completed suicides, but for them there is a simple solution: a physical barrier such as a tall railing at a jump site.

The final chapter, "Ending Suicide," describes the ultimate goal of this book. My intention is to end suicides, not just prevent them. There is a difference. Clinicians and other mental health professionals prevent suicides one patient at a time, but only as a society can we actually end them. Effectively ending suicides in many parts of the United States and eventually across the country might seem impossible, but it isn't. Suicide is the most preventable form of death. Moreover, a large, health maintenance organization in Detroit has shown the way.

In 2001, the Behavioral Health Services division of the Henry Ford Health System implemented what many people considered to be a radical program. Prior to that time, the suicide rate among patients enrolled in the system was seven times the national average. Four years after the program was begun, however, patient suicides had dropped by 75 percent.[7] That was good, but not good enough. The goal was perfection—zero suicides. And Henry Ford achieved it. In 2009, when *JAMA*, the *Journal of the American Medical Association*, reported on the program, there hadn't been a single suicide at Henry Ford in two and a half years.[8]

That success was the inspiration for the Zero Suicide movement. This book builds on that movement by detailing what every facet of society—individuals, clergy, schools, businesses, elected officials, the military, and others—can do to end suicides.

Some people assume that suicides can't be prevented, much less ended. They assume that if someone wants to die by suicide, it might be possible to stop him or her initially, but sooner or later the person will find a way to do it. This assumption is an enabling one. It enables the rest of us to be passive, and that is at the heart of the problem. Answers exist, but often people aren't willing to pursue them. It's time—past time—that we started.

PART I

UNDERSTANDING SUICIDE

CHAPTER 1

Fiction vs. Fact

MANY WELL-KNOWN WRITERS HAVE DIED BY SUICIDE—Ernest Hemingway, Jack London, Sylvia Plath, Virginia Woolf, Anne Sexton, Jerzy Kosiński, David Foster Wallace, Richard Brautigan, Iris Chang, Stefan Zweig, Arthur Koestler, Hunter S. Thompson, Primo Levi, Yukio Mishima, and Nobel laureate Yasunari Kawabata, to name a few. Many artists, musicians, and actors have too—Mark Rothko, Diane Arbus, Vincent Van Gogh, Abbie Hoffman, Phil Ochs, Kurt Cobain, Naomi Judd, Marilyn Monroe, Robin Williams, Freddy Prinze, Spalding Gray, one-time Superman George Reeves, and Edwin Pearce Christy of the Christy Minstrels.

Numerous athletes have joined them. The list includes All-Pro football players Junior Seau, Mike Webster, and Jim Tyrer, "Miracle on Ice" hockey star Mark Pavelich, Olympic beach volleyball medalist Mike Whitmarsh, Olympic freestyle skiing medalist Jeret Peterson, Olympic women's cycling medalist Kelly Catlin, pro golfer Erica Blasberg, Cy Young Award winner Mike Flanagan, Yankees pitcher Hideki Irabu, and Angels pitcher Donnie Moore.

Fashion designer Kate Spade, chef and food critic Anthony Bourdain, George Eastman, founder of Eastman Kodak, Ray Raymond, who founded Victoria's Secret, and Rudolf Diesel, who invented the diesel engine, also killed themselves. So too did former Senate majority leader William Knowland, former secretary of defense James Forrestal, Deputy White House counsel Vince Foster, and Democratic Party fundraiser Duane Garrett. Sigmund Freud, Bruno Bettelheim, Meriwether Lewis, Socrates, and scientist and mathematician Alan Turing were victims of suicide as well.

Two of Bing Crosby's sons died by suicide, as did the sons of Gregory Peck, Willie Nelson, James Arness, Marie Osmond, Mia Farrow, Carroll O'Connor, Charles Boyer, Louis Jourdan, Ray Milland, Danielle Steel, Tony Dungy, Judy Collins, and Lisa Marie Presley. The daughters of Winston Churchill, Marlon Brando, Art Linkletter, and Burt Bacharach and Angie Dickinson also killed themselves. Other suicide victims include the mothers of Drew Brees and Jane and Peter Fonda (Henry Fonda's wife), the fathers of Ted Turner, Archie Manning, and Chesley Sullenberger, the spouses of Robert F. Kennedy Jr., Katharine Graham, Bill Bixby, and Isadora Duncan, the longtime girlfriend of Mick Jagger, the sisters of David Sedaris and Charlotte Rampling, the half-sister of Julia Roberts, and Anderson Cooper's brother (Gloria Vanderbilt's younger son).

Some families have experienced multiple generations of suicide. Not only did Sylvia Plath kill herself but so did Plath's mother and son. Actress Mariette Hartley's father, uncle, and cousin all died by suicide. Ernest Hemingway's father killed himself, as did two siblings (one of whom found Ernest's body),[1] plus granddaughter and model Margaux Hemingway.

According to the Centers for Disease Control and Prevention (CDC), the suicide rate in the United States has increased by 30 percent over the past twenty years, to an all-time high of 49,499 in 2022. Chapter 3 analyzes the data by age, gender, geographic area, ethnicity, day of the week, month of the year, and even weather, but what is important to remember is that suicide is the tenth leading cause of death overall and second among people aged 25 to 44.[2]

According to the federal Substance Abuse and Mental Health Services Administration, more than 1.1 million Americans attempt suicide each year. More than 2.2 million Americans make a suicide plan. More than 8.4 million Americans seriously consider suicide.[3] According to a 2015 study published in the research journal *Suicide and Life-Threatening Behavior*, the national cost of suicide and suicide attempts in 2013, the most recent year for which data were available, was $58.4 billion. Most of this cost (97 percent) was indirect, the result of lost productivity, but the direct cost, primarily for medical treatment, was $1.7 billion.[4] Given the continuing increase in suicides since then and the rising cost of health care, it's reasonable to assume that the cost is at least $2 billion annually today, and probably more.

In light of these statistics, it's natural to ask how something so tragic that happens so frequently can be so misunderstood. Why don't we as a society know more about suicide? The answer lies in an examination of fiction and facts.

Fiction 1: People Who Are Suicidal Want to Die

Many people are ambivalent when it comes to suicide. Often they leave it up to others or fate to decide the outcome.

A young man, heavily medicated and despondent, walks on the pedestrian side of the Golden Gate Bridge. "If one person smiles at me," he writes in a note that he leaves on his dresser, "I won't jump." The coroner finds the note in the man's sparsely furnished apartment after his suicide.[5]

Behind the closed door of her bedroom, a teenage girl swallows a handful of pills. She doesn't know whether it's a lethal amount but will accept whatever happens because she is tired of hurting. If someone finds her in time, she will wake up in a hospital bed, no better off than she was before, but no worse off either. If she doesn't wake up, her pain will be over.

Several boys play Russian roulette with a loaded gun that one boy has stolen from his father. It's a daring game of chance with potentially fatal consequences. None of the boys is particularly eager to die, but they have been sharing a bottle, come from broken homes, face futures that appear bleak, and don't see much point to living.

In 1975 David Rosen, a San Francisco psychiatrist, interviewed six survivors of a Golden Gate Bridge jump. Rosen admitted that it was a small sample, but then few people have lived after leaping from the bridge. Rosen found that the six had several things in common. Each was young—under 30 and in most cases closer to 20. Each hit the water feet first and at a slight angle, so that their bodies arced back to the surface, which prevented them from drowning. Most important of all, each one said that he or she wanted to live as soon as they went over the side. Moreover, they didn't have a plan B; it was the Golden Gate Bridge or nothing.[6]

Thorton McKay jumped from the bridge on December 27, 2022—two days after Christmas and nine days after his twenty-third birthday. He too survived, despite puncturing a lung, tearing his esophagus, and breaking two vertebrae in his back. He was in the hospital for a month, and soon after he was released he went to Coast Guard Station Golden Gate and personally thanked some of the crew members who had rescued him. "I look back on that, and man, that's the worst, darkest feeling I was ever in," he said afterward. Childhood trauma, depression, and bipolar disorder had led him to take a bus to the bridge, where, despite a fear of heights and drowning, he jumped without hesitation. "I'm glad where I'm at," he says now. "I'm glad I get a second opportunity."[7]

Thinking that people want to die is a way of writing them off before it happens, as if they merit no further consideration. "Jump!" some observers shout to the man perched on the ledge of a tall building. Get it over with. It's a cruel thing to say, and something that doubtless wouldn't be said if the man were someone they knew and cared about. The fact that he is a stranger makes what happens to him irrelevant to those in the crowd. They share a degree of fascination at his plight and wonder what it was that led him to the ledge, but that is all.

Thinking that people want to die also serves as justification for doing nothing about it. If a person believes that someone who is suicidal can't be talked out of it, or that it's their life and they can do whatever they want with it—including ending it—then prevention seems pointless. Just go about your business and let others worry about theirs.

Anytime life becomes unbearable, death is an option. This doesn't mean that a person willingly chooses to die, however. Even people who have been diagnosed with a terminal illness rarely resort to suicide.[8] Humans aren't wired that way. From an early age, we are taught to resist death as long as possible. "It beats the alternative" is a common remark when someone comments on the tribulations of aging. Life may be challenging, but it's better than dying.

If we are hurting, we want the pain to go away, and the sharper and deeper it is the more we want to be free of it. Should it get really bad, when living another day is the worst thing imaginable, death may seem to be not only a viable alternative but the only option. This doesn't mean that people want to die, though. Rather, they don't want to live, at least as they are living now. Anything, even death, is thought to be better.

Fiction 2: Suicidal People Resort to Any Means Possible

Most adults who are suicidal plan their death. They think about how they want to do it, where, and when. The degree of planning is a strong indicator of the risk. The more concrete a person's plan, the more likely they are to implement it. Adolescents are prone to impulsiveness, but adults tend to think about things before they act. This is why the first step for helpers is to assess the risk and determine whether an attempt is imminent.

In terms of how to do it, there are myriad means—gun, knife, rope, pills, car, poisons, or jumping. In today's world, people have access to multiple means, so it becomes a matter of choice. Guns are lethal, but they leave a mess. The thought of cutting themselves is abhorrent to some people, while others fear asphyxiation. Pills and carbon monoxide poisoning take longer and leave open the possibility of intervention. In other words, even though people kill themselves in various ways, most have a preferred method.

The decision involves two questions: will it be quick, and will it be painless? Individuals intent on suicide don't want a lingering death. They want life over with now. In addition, they don't want to experience any more pain than they are experiencing already. That pain is what drove them to this point, and the thought of adding to it is unthinkable.

Two other questions sometimes enter into the equation as well: is death virtually guaranteed, and who will find one's body? Some means are more lethal than others. A person is much more likely to die from a gunshot wound than from a drug overdose. Many people survive drug overdoses, but few people survive a bullet in the head. Similarly, cutting one's wrists isn't the easiest thing to do, and it isn't nearly as deadly as jumping from a high bridge, a tall building, or a cliff.

For individuals who are committed to dying and have no ambivalence about it, who don't want others to know, don't display any obvious warning signs, and don't want to be saved, the chosen means is one for which the odds overwhelmingly favor death. This still can mean a jump, but more likely it means a firearm. One woman who lived in San Francisco did both—she jumped from the Golden Gate Bridge and shot herself in the head on the way down, not only ensuring that she would die but avoiding the pain of hitting the water.

This was known after the fact because she said as much in a note that she left behind.[9]

Bridges are popular for some suicidal people because there isn't a death scene for loved ones to discover. Individuals either sink into oblivion, never to be seen again, or their body is recovered by first responders—police officers, paramedics, or the Coast Guard—who deliver it to a coroner. Either way, family members are spared a gruesome cleanup. Some suicidal people kill themselves in remote locations, such as parks, so that family members don't find their remains. Others rent hotel rooms for the same reason—so that strangers rather than loved ones deal with the immediate aftermath.

The bottom line is that people who plan their death think about the means. They don't make a haphazard attempt but rather decide in advance how they are going to do it, taking whatever steps are necessary—gaining access to a firearm and ammunition, stockpiling medications, learning how to tie a hangman's knot, knowing how to direct a car's exhaust into the sealed cabin of the vehicle, or researching whether a potential jump site has a suicide barrier.

Once they decide on the means and the location, they settle on a date. In many instances this isn't arbitrary. Often an anniversary—of a marriage, a divorce, a birthday, a death—is chosen because of its special meaning. This is why helpers pay attention to anniversaries, and why part of their safety planning is focused on getting suicidal people past these dates. A person still may attempt suicide—there are no guarantees that the risk has ended—but at least the helper has bought time. In suicide prevention, buying time can be everything.

Fiction 3: People Who Talk about Suicide Won't Really Do It

Before attempting suicide, many individuals make direct statements about their intention to end their life or less direct comments to the effect that they have nothing to live for, that they might as well be dead, or that their family and friends will be better off without them. Often these comments produce little or no reaction because the person hearing them either doesn't take them seriously or doesn't want to believe them.

After a death by suicide, family members and friends frequently recall recent conversations they had with the deceased, conversations in which the person voiced thoughts that, in retrospect, were ominous. Unfortunately, that realization is too late. Any reference to suicide should be taken seriously. It's a call for help, perhaps the only one that a suicidal person makes. If no one acts on it, the message is that no one cares.

When someone has a drinking problem or a drug problem, others offer advice or at least talk about it. The same isn't true with suicide. People fear the conversation because they don't know what to say to someone who is thinking seriously about suicide. As a result, family members and friends say nothing, which usually is worse than anything they could have said. It causes a suicidal person to stop confiding in them and to withdraw even more.

Sometimes people are silent because they believe that if they mention suicide, they will plant the idea in someone's mind when it wasn't there before. We have public campaigns against smoking and drunk driving, though, and few people worry that these campaigns lead individuals to engage in a targeted behavior when they didn't before.

At one time, when I talked frequently to groups of parents about youth suicide, someone voiced this concern. In the beginning I said that this just wasn't true, that raising the subject of suicide and in fact asking someone about it can be an act of compassion. It fosters open and honest communication between loved ones and encourages people to seek help. After a while, though, I wasn't convinced that this message was getting through. People heard it, but I wasn't sure they truly believed it. That was when I borrowed an idea from Eve Meyer, the longtime executive director of San Francisco Suicide

Prevention. "Are you thinking about killing yourself?" I asked the person. Usually he or she recoiled in horror and said, "Definitely not." I nodded and continued to talk for a few more minutes. At some point I returned to the person who had asked the question and said, "Are you thinking about killing yourself now?" Again, the person was taken aback and said, emphatically, no. This time, though, my message got through.

A person who expresses suicidal thoughts has been contemplating suicide well before saying anything. Questioning him or her about it isn't planting the notion; it's showing them that you're concerned and are willing to listen. According to researchers at Columbia University, asking about suicide doesn't put the idea in a young person's head. On the contrary, screening students for suicidal ideation and planning "is a safe component of youth suicide prevention efforts," researchers concluded.[10]

Fiction 4: People Who Are Suicidal
Are Suicidal Forever

Individuals who have seriously considered killing themselves and possibly attempted it don't think about suicide every waking moment. The desire to die, to be free of pain and suffering, comes and goes. It may never disappear entirely, but nor is it foremost in a person's mind all the time.

According to the T. H. Chan Harvard School of Public Health, 90 percent of people who survive a suicide attempt don't go on to kill themselves. "Suicidal crises are often short-lived, even if there may be underlying, more chronic risk factors present that give rise to these crises," the school reports.[11] A review in the *British Journal of Psychiatry* of ninety studies that followed over time people who had received medical care following a suicide attempt reported similar findings. Only 7 percent of attempters eventually died by suicide.[12] The fact is that most people who survive an attempt find reasons to live. It might be family or friends, or it might be a vow to do something positive with their remaining years in gratitude for being given a second chance.

Kevin Hines is one of the few survivors of a Golden Gate Bridge jump. In 2000 he was 19 years old, distraught, and battling inner demons. He took a bus to the bridge and for more than twenty minutes paced the span, contemplating whether to jump. All the while tears streamed down his face as he considered the enormity of the decision and how his parents would feel when they heard the news.

Oblivious to his pain, a young woman with a camera and a German accent asked him to take her picture on the bridge. Hines took the picture, then said to himself, "That's it. No one cares about me."[13] He sprinted to the four-foot-tall railing and threw himself over the side.

Instantly, he regretted it. As soon as he jumped, he wanted to live.

As he was hurtling toward the water head first at seventy-five miles per hour, Hines somehow managed in the four seconds of his fall to right himself so that he entered the water feet first, giving him the best chance to survive. Other factors then came into play: he was able to push himself back to the surface despite plunging deeply and suffering serious injuries, his jump was witnessed, the Coast Guard was contacted immediately, a boat got to the scene quickly and pulled him from the water, and he was taken by ambulance to San Francisco General Hospital, where doctors treated him successfully for hypothermia, broken bones, and damaged organs. This confluence of events, plus the fact that he was young and in good physical shape, saved his life.

During his rehabilitation, a hospital chaplain suggested to Hines that talking to others about his depression and jump might help in the healing process. A middle school invited him to speak, and afterward Hines received thank-you letters from 120 students, 6 of whom said that they too had been dealing with suicidal thoughts.[14]

Since then Hines has become the most visible advocate for a suicide barrier on the Golden Gate Bridge. He has told his story hundreds of times to students, reporters, bridge district officials, and others. More recently, he wrote a book about it (*Cracked, not Broken: Surviving and Thriving after a Suicide Attempt*) and produced a documentary movie (*Suicide: The Ripple Effect*). Today he travels the world speaking with a two-part message. The first part is that suicide can be prevented, and one way to do it is to restrict easy access to lethal means such as physical barriers at jump sites. The second part is that while living with a mental illness is challenging, it doesn't have to be defining. Spreading his message has become Hines's calling, and despite dealing with his own mental health issues and physical disabilities, the latter due to his fall, he has worked hard to become an articulate and effective spokesperson.

For the first five years after his jump, Hines went to the Golden Gate Bridge every year on September 24. In addition to being the anniversary of his jump, in his mind it was also the anniversary of his rebirth. He would walk to the exact spot where he had leaped and look down at the dark water 220 feet below. He didn't have thoughts of suicide anymore, but he didn't want to forget that day either. It has shaped every moment of his life since.

Fiction 5: Once a Suicidal Crisis Passes, the Danger Is Over

Fiction 5 is the opposite of the previous fiction. It assumes that after a person has been hospitalized for a suicide attempt and then released, the danger has diminished. In fact, the opposite is true. One study found that for men the risk of suicide is 102 times greater in the first week after discharge from a psychiatric hospital for a suicide attempt, while for women it's 256 times greater.[15] One reason for this is the mistaken belief that when a person is discharged, doctors and nurses have dealt with the problem and loved ones can relax. On the contrary, loved ones need to get the person into longer-term care, such as counseling, in order to deal with root causes.

According to the federal Substance Abuse and Mental Health Services Administration, 77 percent of individuals who have died by suicide visited their primary care physician within the past year, 45 percent within the past month. Ten percent were discharged from a hospital within the past sixty days.[16] The National Institutes of Health reports that 38 percent of individuals who have attempted suicide visited a health care provider—primary care, specialty care, or emergency department—within the week prior to their attempt. Nearly all—95 percent—visited a health care provider within the preceding year.[17]

What this means is that people see doctors fairly frequently, but these visits have little or nothing to do with suicide prevention, mainly because the subject of suicide doesn't come up. People generally are much more comfortable admitting to a physical problem than to a psychological one—because of the stigma of mental illness—and physicians aren't trained to ask. As a result, an opportunity is missed.

Related to this is the phenomenon whereby, after a prolonged period of depression, suicidal people exhibit elevated mood swings, leading others to think that the danger has passed or at least subsided. The upbeat attitude is misinterpreted as a sign that people are getting better, that they are feeling more optimistic about life. In fact, they are upbeat for an entirely different reason: they have made the decision to die. They have taken control of their lives after feeling out of control and believe that the end to their pain and suffering is near.

Fiction 6: Suicide Is an Impulsive Act

The notion that suicide is an impulsive act appears to have empirical support. For example, in 2001 researchers at the University of

Houston studied 153 people who had survived a suicide attempt. They found that 87 percent of these individuals had thought about suicide for fewer than eight hours before acting. For 70 percent, the attempt occurred within one hour of making the decision. Most astonishing of all, 24 percent said that they had attempted suicide within *five minutes* of deciding to kill themselves.[18] In other words, the interval between thinking about suicide and making an attempt was only an hour for most members of the group, and for one out of four people almost no time elapsed between the impulse to kill themselves and the attempt.

Researchers in Australia who interviewed people in an emergency room shortly after they had been admitted following a suicide attempt reached a similar conclusion. Half the people said that they had thought about killing themselves for no more than ten minutes before acting, and another 16 percent said that the time period had been less than thirty minutes.[19]

Studies like these lend credence to the belief that suicide is impulsive. Indeed, one psychiatrist, writing in the *New York Times*, cited them in arguing that mental health providers perpetuate the false narrative of suicide being a planned act. Much broader factors, she said, in particular "poverty, homelessness, and the accompanying exposure to trauma, crime, and drugs, need to be addressed first. Until then, suicide prevention offers only 'empty promises.'"[20]

Studies like those at the University of Houston and in Australia have two significant flaws, however. First, they are based on self-reports, which often are unreliable. A person whose judgment is impaired because of a mental disorder, alcohol, drugs, intense psychological pain, or even a lack of sleep isn't always able to describe accurately what he or she was thinking or feeling in the moment. In the Australian study, 29 percent of participants said that they had been drinking at the time of their attempt, and nearly everyone in this subgroup—93 percent—reported the interval between the time that they thought about killing themselves and the time of their attempt as being ten minutes at most. Second, researchers didn't delve into participants' pasts to discover whether they had ever contemplated suicide before. An attempt that might have seemed like a spur-of-the-moment decision could have been the result of days, weeks, months, or even years of suicidal ideation and tentative planning.

The live, on-air suicide of TV news reporter Christine Chubbuck in Florida in 1974—the subject of two movies in 2016—struck many people as impulsive. Not her family, though. The 29-year-old woman had been suicidal for years and had made one previous attempt, by overdosing. This time, after Christine bought a gun, she told a colleague at work that she might shoot herself on the air, but he thought she was joking. Several weeks earlier, her news director had given her permission to research a story on suicide. In an interview with a police officer she had asked what was the surest way to kill oneself. He had answered that it was a gunshot to the head, specifically to the back of the head rather than the temple.

On the fateful day, Chubbuck reported a shooting in a restaurant, then said, "In keeping with Channel 40's policy of bringing you the latest in blood and guts, and in living color, you are going to see another first—an attempted suicide." She then took the gun from her purse, shot herself in the back of the head, and died fourteen hours later in a hospital. Afterward, people found the copy she had written with those words on it, plus her script for a staff person to read on air immediately following the incident in which her condition was reported as "critical."

In literature there are numerous instances of characters who kill themselves in an impetuous manner, with Anna Karenina throwing herself under the wheels of a train being the prime example. The use of impulsivity by writers like Tolstoy, Shakespeare, and others for narrative effect in describing suicides is misleading. "This is simply not how it works in the real world," says Thomas Joiner, a noted suicide expert whose own father died by suicide, "else there would be millions more suicides per year as people glance at knives and trains and the like."[21]

For some people—mainly adolescents—suicide can be impulsive;[22] however most individuals plan their death. They procure the means, decide on a date and location, then put their plan into action. "The idea that suicidal acts come out of the blue undermines the attempts to study, assess, treat, and prevent them," Joiner says. "Suicide is tractable, and we owe it to the memories of those who have died already and to those who are at risk in the future to make it more so."[23]

Fiction 7: Homicides Are a Bigger Problem than Suicides

In the beginning of this chapter I named nearly one hundred well-known people who have killed themselves or lost children, parents, spouses, siblings, or other loved ones to suicide. Contrast that with the number of famous people who have been murdered. Other than political figures who have been assassinated, I can name only four—John Lennon, the rapper Tupac Shakur, the Mexican American singer Selena, and the zoologist Dian Fossey. Several high-profile people, such as actress Natalie Wood, activist Karen Silkwood, and Teamsters president Jimmy Hoffa, died under questionable circumstances, but their deaths have never been confirmed as homicides. Actress Sharon Tate, who was murdered by Charles Manson and his gang, is remembered more because of her murder than because of her movie career. The same is even truer for child model JonBenet Ramsey, whose murder remains a mystery but who otherwise would be unknown by most people.

In small communities murders receive widespread attention, for good reason: they are relatively rare, and many people know the victim. Even in large cities, however, where murders are frequent and the victims tend to be strangers, most homicides receive press attention. "If it bleeds, it leads" isn't an empty phrase but rather one that means greater sales for media outlets that report stories filled with violence and bloodshed.

The opposite is true when it comes to suicides. People don't want to read about them, so that media coverage minimal to nonexistent. The social prohibition that keeps people from talking about suicide—unless a well-known figure is involved—also keeps the press from covering it. Stephen Dubner, the host of the podcast *Freakonomics*, says that "murder represents a fractured promise within our social contract, and it's got an obvious villain. Suicide represents—well, what does it represent? It's hard to say. It carries such a strong taboo that most of us just don't discuss it."[24]

Given this cloak of silence, it's not surprising that the public assumes that homicides occur more frequently than suicides. In fact, though, it's the opposite. The number of people who kill themselves in the United States is more than double the number who are murdered (an average of 48,000 suicides per year in recent years, compared with 20,000 homicides per year).

That said, there are three places in the country where the homicide rate is higher than the suicide rate—Louisiana, Maryland, and the District of Columbia. Dubner, on *Freakonomics*, theorized that this anomaly is due to the fact that all three places have a high percentage of African Americans, who he said "are only about half as likely to kill themselves as whites. When it comes to murder, meanwhile, African-Americans are nearly six times more likely than whites to die."[25]

The disparity in news coverage is one reason why the misperception exists that homicides are more frequent than suicides. There is another reason, however: television. "The average American will watch more TV by the time he is six than he will spend talking to his father for the rest of his life," writes George Howe Colt. "By the time he graduates from high school, he will have logged 20,000 hours in front of the TV, compared with 11,000 hours in the classroom."[26] By age 18, Colt says, the average person will have witnessed 40,000 TV murders, compared with 800 TV suicides.[27] The difference between the number of depicted homicides and the number of depicted suicides, with the former being fifty times greater than the latter, perpetuates the belief that murder is more common than suicide.

Advocates of commonsense gun laws often cite the number of firearm deaths in the United States—48,000 in 2022—as a reason for tougher restrictions on the sale and distribution of guns. Rarely, though, do they or others note that more than half of all firearm deaths in this country are the result of suicides, not homicides.[28] Personally, I'm in favor of anything that makes procuring a gun harder, but it bothers me when suicide is removed from the equation. I understand why this is the case—people will be less moved to act if suicide is mentioned, and 20,000 homicide deaths per year from firearms doesn't have the same impact as 48,000 firearm deaths—but it serves as another way of keeping suicide underreported and in the shadows.

Fiction 8: Most Religions and Cultures Consider Suicide a Sin

Christianity, Judaism, and Islam once took harsh positions when it came to suicide. The Catholic Church considered suicide to be the work of the devil and didn't permit memorial services or burial on church grounds for anyone who died by suicide. The belief was that God had granted the miracle of life, and stopping something that he had started was a sin. Among Jews, attitudes were similar. Suicide was a rebellion against God, and rabbis wouldn't observe mourning rites. In Islam, Muhammad proclaimed that suicide victims were denied paradise and would spend eternity in hell.

These attitudes have softened in recent years, partly owing to a greater understanding about why people kill themselves and partly because people are more aware of the role that mental illness plays. The result is a nuanced acceptance that is perhaps most noticeable in the *Catechism of the Catholic Church.*

Paragraph 2281 of the *Catechism* states, "Suicide contradicts the natural inclination of the human being to preserve and perpetuate his life. It is gravely contrary to the just love of self. It likewise offends love of neighbor because it unjustly breaks the ties of solidarity with family, nation, and other human societies to which we continue to have obligations. Suicide is contrary to the love for the living God."

The next paragraph starts in much the same vein. "If suicide is committed with the intention of setting an example, especially to the young, it also takes on the gravity of scandal." Then it addresses the subject of assisted suicide: "Voluntary co-operation in suicide is contrary to the moral law." After that it equivocates: "Grave psychological disturbances, anguish, or grave fear of hardship, suffering, or torture can diminish the responsibility of the one committing suicide."

Paragraph 2283 goes further, stating, "We should not despair of the eternal salvation of persons who have taken their own lives. By ways unknown to him alone, God can provide the opportunity for salutary repentance. The Church prays for persons who have taken their own lives."[29] In other words, God can have mercy on people who kill themselves, which means that suicide isn't a sin. Previous practices that pertained to memorializing and burying suicide victims have changed as a result, to the point where funeral masses for suicide deaths are permitted, as is burial on church grounds.

In the Orthodox Church, suicide is considered to be a rejection of God's gift of physical life, and a Christian burial is often—but not always—denied. Exceptions are made if information comes to light, verified by a physician, that a person suffered from a mental illness or severe emotional stress. Similarly, among Mormons suicide is viewed as wrong; however, factors such as motive and character may be taken into account. The actions of an individual, while not condoned, can be absolved to some extent.

As for Jews who end up taking their lives, they now receive all rites of mourning because their actions are considered the result of temporary insanity caused by depression. Although frowned upon as a practice, suicide is excused because the very act proves that the person wasn't in his or her right frame of mind. Assisting in a suicide is forbidden, however.

For people of Islamic faith, whether a suicide victim goes to heaven or hell is in God's hands, as is everything else. A line in the Qur'an states, "Do not kill yourselves, surely God is most Merciful to you."[30] Suicidal terrorists who believe that their acts will hasten entry to paradise are thought to interpret traditional Islamic teachings in a perverse and self-serving manner, although according to the Pew Research Center, a minority of Muslims support suicidal martyrdom to varying degrees.[31]

Culturally, some forms of suicide may be condoned. In India, for instance, suttee, the act of a Hindu woman throwing herself onto her husband's funeral pyre to prove her devotion to him, continues in some areas today even though the British government banned it in 1829. In some Asian countries the stigma of suicide is so strong that *mental illness* literally translates as "crazy illness." People readily seek treatment from doctors for physical injuries, but the closest they come to admitting any kind of mental illness is to complain of headaches.

Despite religious dogma that discourages suicide, there is little empirical evidence that one's religious beliefs do much to keep one from killing oneself. One challenge is that there are many dimensions to religion,[32] from loosely subscribing to a particular doctrine and attending religious services infrequently or rarely to being devout, wholly invested and observant, and regularly attending services. If asked, congregants might describe themselves one way and act differently in practice, making the extent of their beliefs hard to measure. Similarly, there are different dimensions to suicide, from ideation and planning to attempt and completion, and someone may downplay the extent to which he or she has contemplated suicide—or not admit to it at all. A third variable is that some religions tend to attract certain cultural groups that are more socially isolated than other groups and potentially at greater risk of suicide because of their lack of connectedness outside the church.

Fiction 9: Humans Are the Only Animals Who Die by Suicide

Some people consider suicide to be unique to humans. If pressed, they may accede to the common image of lemmings marching in a line off a cliff, but in their minds that is the only example in the animal kingdom. Ironically, most scientists don't consider lemmings' behavior to be suicidal. Lemmings migrate en masse when their source of food is depleted and sometimes end up on land that is high above a body of water. Pressed to feed themselves, and pushed by the crowding of others, they jump and often don't survive the fall. Their deaths are considered accidental rather than intentional, though, the more so because lemmings can swim.

Other species do engage in intentional self-sacrifice, which is one way to describe suicide. Male fire ants and male honeybees die in the course of mating. The same is true of Australian redback spiders and pea aphids. In passing on their genes during the reproductive process, they sustain the group.

Additional examples are subject to debate. We know that animals, like humans, can suffer from depression. Monkeys are known to grieve when a companion dies, and some dogs refuse to eat after their owner's death. Is that suicide? Are dogs and other nonhuman species able to self-reflect and develop the capacity to intentionally kill themselves out of grief or despair? We don't know.

In 2016 *BBC News* reported that a captive bear at a bear farm in China smothered her male cub and then killed herself. "This followed an extremely painful injection of a catheter into the bear cub's abdomen to extract bile," the BBC said, "which is sometimes used in Chinese medicine. Newspaper reports suggested that the mother bear killed her son to prevent more years of torture," then took her own life.[33]

Also in 2016, a video shot at SeaWorld's Tenerife water park in the Canary Islands went viral after an orca born in the wild beached itself on the side of her tank for ten minutes in what some people theorized was a suicide attempt. Inasmuch as SeaWorld orcas live in small, unnatural environments for a prolonged period of time, it's possible that deliberate self-injurious behavior like this is a response to their imprisonment. That may be a humanistic interpretation, however, as is the notion that the orca might have been trying to escape.

On occasion, whales strand themselves on a beach in what could be construed as mass suicide. Another explanation, however, is that whales form social groups and could be following a sick individual into shallow water where it feels safer, in the process becoming stranded.

Barbara King, of the College of William & Mary in Virginia, has written about animal grief and suicide. She says that we are not at a point where we can read an animal's mind. "We can look at their visible behavior as we do with grief, but we cannot look at what amounts to harm that comes to an animal and assess whether it's intended or not intended."[34]

Ancient Greeks believed they knew the answer. Claudius Aelian, a second-century Greek scholar, noted twenty-one instances of what he claimed were animal suicides, including a dolphin that let itself be captured and an eagle that "sacrificed itself by combustion on the pyre of its dead master."[35] Aristotle cited the example of a stallion that threw itself over a cliff after it became apparent that the horse, like Oedipus, had mated with his own mother unknowingly.[36]

In later years, similar instances of perceived animal suicide have been cited, sometimes by animal rights activists seeking to ascribe human emotions to animals as a way of protecting them. Again, though, science hasn't proved whether this is real or imagined. The most we can say is that it's possible and more study is needed.

Fiction 10: Suicide Ends the Pain

It's true that when people die by suicide, their pain ends. Whether they believe in reincarnation and life everlasting or that their soul and spirit expire at the same time that their heart stops pumping, they suffer no longer. The pain isn't over, though, for everyone who loves them. In many respects it's just beginning. This is because suicide transfers the pain from the dead to the living, who carry it with them until they too die—sometimes by suicide. The noted suicide expert Edwin Shneidman said that a person who dies by suicide "puts his psychological skeletons in the survivor's emotional basket."[37]

One person's suicide can leave those who follow at greater risk for the same kind of self-destructive behavior. In this respect suicide is similar to child abuse and domestic violence, which also can be passed down through generations. Breaking the cycle isn't easy. There is a significant difference, though. Child abuse and domestic violence are committed predominantly by males, with females being the primary victims. Suicide, by contrast, affects both genders more or less equally. More males die by suicide than females, but more females attempt suicide than males. It's a legacy that needs to end.

CHAPTER 2

The Proverbial Question

WHENEVER SOMEONE DIES BY SUICIDE, PEOPLE ASK WHY. Why did he or she do it? It was the question asked in *Time* magazine after actor-comedian Robin Williams killed himself.[1] It's the focus of Eric Marcus's book *Why Suicide?* College quarterback Tyler Hilinski took his life four months after being carried off the field by delirious Washington State fans following his team's triple overtime victory over Boise State, prompting a long article in *Sports Illustrated* titled "The Search for Why."[2]

Often there isn't an answer, or at least there isn't an answer that seems to make sense. Suicidal behavior is complex, and rarely is it attributable to one reason. In *November of the Soul: The Enigma of Suicide* George Howe Colt writes, "While it is often said that suicide may be committed by 12 different people for 12 different reasons, it may be just as true to say that one person may choose death for 12 different reasons or 100 different reasons—psychological, sociological, and biological factors that finally tighten around one place and time like a knot."[3] A man who kills himself in response to voices that are urging him to do so, says Colt, is different from a man who is terminally ill, in constant pain, and "has had enough of life." A woman who has been depressed for many years, periodically contemplating suicide, is different from a teenage girl who is a victim of cyberbullying and leaps from a bridge.

In his landmark book about suicide, *Man Against Himself*, published in 1938, Karl Menninger hypothesizes about a wealthy man who kills himself. In the aftermath of his death, people discover that his investments have failed, leaving him penniless, although his family is cared for by a life insurance policy that enables them to avoid destitution. "The problem and its solution, then, seem simple and obvious enough," Menninger writes. "A man has bravely faced ruin in a way that benefits his dependents."

But wait, Menninger says. "Why should we begin our interpretations only at this late point in such a man's life, the point at which he loses his wealth? Shall we not seek to discover how it came about that he lost it? And even more pertinently, shall we not inquire how he made it, why he was driven to amass money, and what means he used to gratify his compulsion, what unconscious and perhaps also conscious guilt feelings were associated with it and with the sacrifices and penalties its acquisition cost him and his family?"

Menninger goes on to say that the vast majority of people who have money and lose it don't kill themselves, so even knowing the answers to the above questions doesn't necessarily mean that anyone has a better understanding of someone's motives. He concludes that "all we can really see from such a case is how difficult and complex the problem becomes as soon as we take more than a superficial glance at the circumstances."[4]

The simplest and most basic explanation of suicide is found in Ernest Hemingway's short story "Indian Camp." Nick Adams's father is a doctor. As he is delivering a woman's baby, her husband, who is in the same room, cuts his throat. Nick witnesses the horror, and afterward he asks his father why the Indian killed himself. His father replies, "I don't know, Nick. He couldn't stand things, I guess."[5]

It's reasonable to think that a suicide note provides the answer, or at least a telltale clue. Generally this isn't the case, however. For one thing, only 30 percent of suicide victims leave a note. Most do not.[6] Few members of the general public have ever seen a suicide note. Second, there aren't any rules about what one should include in the note or even whom the note should be addressed to. Does a person ask for forgiveness from loved ones, cite reasons of rejection and isolation in order to hurt others, or provide instructions about money and insurance or the disposal of the deceased's remains? Third, the contents of notes left may be meager, lacking the passion and desperation usually associated with suicide. Often the note appears to be an afterthought.

Here are a few samples of notes left by persons who died by jumping off the Golden Gate Bridge:

"Spent all day yesterday walking around San Francisco deciding what to do. This is the only thing I could do with all the trouble I have caused. Please remember I loved you very much. Take the insurance money and settle the bills."

"Dear Mother, everything I have done has been a lie. Everything Dad did was a lie. I am going to do away with myself before I do further harm to people."

"Honey, I know that anything I have done or do is all on myself. Something was and is wrong with my makeup and there is not anything that anyone can do about it. I love you. Goodbye."[7]

Since a person's last words usually fail to enlighten, even in the rare instances when they form a long soliloquy, it is left to researchers to explain. The challenge is that while suicide is a universal phenomenon, affecting people of all ages, starting as young as 10, all ethnicities, all cultures, and all socioeconomic groups, the incidence of suicide varies among nationalities, races, religions, and professions, as well as between men and women. For example, worldwide suicide rates are highest for the elderly, and in every country except China elderly men are at greater risk. In China, though, elderly women have the higher suicide rate. In the United States, elderly white men have the highest rate, especially those living in western states. Seniors of other races, as well as those living in the East, have lower rates. Among youths, Native Americans are most at risk, gay and lesbian teens have elevated rates, and girls attempt suicide more often than boys, though boys have a higher rate. How does one explain the differences?

Physicians and prostitutes have high rates of suicide, but why? Suicides increase during times of economic crisis and decrease during times of national crisis, but why? Far fewer people died by suicide in the United States on February 22, 1980, than on any February 22 in the preceding or following twenty years, but why?

How is it possible to understand mass suicides in cults? Why is suicide associated more frequently with anorexia than with bulimia? Why is self-injury by cutting or piercing a gateway to suicide even though it's rarely intended as a suicidal act?

It's like trying to put together a puzzle when some of the pieces are missing. A person may think that he or she knows what it's supposed to look like, but with empty spaces it's hard to know for certain.

Durkheim and Social Connectedness

In 1897 the French sociologist Émile Durkheim published the first empirical study of suicide. Citing a variety of statistics, Durkheim concluded that (1) suicide is more common among men than among women, although women make more attempts; (2) the elderly are more likely to die by suicide than younger adults or youths; (3) divorced individuals have higher suicide rates than those who are married; and (4) childless adults kill themselves more often than adults who are parents.

Durkheim discounted the influence of mental disorders and psychological distress in explaining suicide. Instead, he believed that suicide rates were related to social factors, in particular to social connectedness. Simply put, when people feel that they are part of a larger group they are less likely to attempt suicide, he said, and when people lack social bonds the likelihood of suicide increases. Working people are more integrated than those who are jobless, Durkheim reasoned, which explains why suicide rates are lower during boom times, when unemployment is down, and higher during recessions, when unemployment is up. He believed that married people, as a rule, tend to be more socially connected than those who are single, divorced, or widowed and therefore are more protected against suicide. Parents with children are even more protected because they tend to be more integrated. Durkheim cautioned, however, that married people living in societies where divorce is common are less protected than those living in societies where divorce is rare.

Geographic mobility is a factor too. Durkheim observed that starting in the latter half of the nineteenth century people began to move farther away from home in order to pursue educational opportunities, employment, and a better way of life. Once on the go, they continued to move, resulting in the disruption of social networks and kin support, which are especially needed during times of crisis. In 2001 the Centers for Disease Control and Prevention reported that one of the more significant predictors of suicide was frequent moves. A 2009 study determined that adolescents aged 11 to 17 who had moved three to five times were twice as likely to attempt suicide as those who had never changed their address.[8]

From the vantage point of current research, there is a lot to critique in Durkheim's work. For one thing, Durkheim considered suicide to be predictable and regular, when it's neither. Suicides occur with predictable regularity, and some populations are at greater risk; however, even in instances where a group such as elderly white men has a high rate, the vast majority of people in the group never contemplate or attempt suicide.

Attributing suicide entirely or even primarily to social factors also is flawed. While some external circumstances, such as divorce, job loss, death of a loved one, gambling debts, or failure in school, can lead to a suicide attempt, they are considered triggers—that is, precipitators—rather than causes. Instead, mental disorders, in particular severe depression that is untreated, play a major role, especially when combined with alcoholism. According to the National Institute of Mental Health, up to 90 percent of the people who die by suicide have a diagnosable mental illness, most often major depression, schizophrenia, or bipolar disorder.[9] This might seem to be contradicted by a 2018 CDC report according to which 54 percent of suicides in the twenty-seven states that use the National Violent Death Reporting System were by people who had no known mental health condition.[10]

The director of NIMH, Joshua Gordon, said that that finding had to be viewed in context, however. "When you do a psychological autopsy and go and look carefully at medical records, and talk to family members of the victims," Gordon said, "90 percent will have evidence of a mental health condition." They may never have been diagnosed for it, however, and as a result may never have received the help they needed.[11] Again, it's important to note that not everyone who is mentally ill is a suicide risk. On the contrary, 95 percent of people with psychiatric disorders don't kill themselves.[12]

Durkheim's definition of suicide—a person's death that results from his or her consciously doing something or avoiding doing something—also is debatable. It includes heroic sacrifice, for instance, and excludes madmen, when today it's the reverse; heroic sacrifice usually isn't viewed as suicide, and the death of a madman—a lone gunman or suicide bomber—is. In addition, Durkheim failed to acknowledge the moral reasons and material interests (such as life insurance benefits) that lead suicide to be underreported. Also, in explaining the disparity between suicide rates by age, Durkheim didn't note that questionable deaths of youths are less likely to be declared suicides because youth suicide carries the greatest stigma, while seniors may have fewer people to care about them or no one around to hide the cause of death.

That said, Durkheim's work still represented a milestone. It demonstrated the value of statistics and methodology, laying the groundwork for future research on suicide. Indeed, the June 2008 issue of *Suicide and Life-Threatening Behavior*, a publication of the American Association of Suicidology and the principal journal in the United States for suicide studies, noted that Durkheim's book, published 111 years earlier, had been cited forty-four times in academic articles from 1997 to 2001, ranking it eighteenth among 8,004 reference sources.[13]

Shneidman and *Psychache*

In 1918, a year after Émile Durkheim died in Paris, Edwin Shneidman was born in Pennsylvania. The juxtaposition of Durkheim's death and Shneidman's birth wasn't exactly a passing of the torch. Shneidman, a psychologist educated in southern California, was more interested in individual behaviors than in social behavior. He made the study of death—thanatology—and in particular suicide the focus of his professional life when, early in his career, he was asked to write condolence letters to the widows of two veterans who had died by suicide. In researching their cases, he discovered a vault at the Los Angeles County Coroner's Office that contained all the suicide notes the office had collected over the years. There was so much unmined data that Shneidman felt as if he had struck gold.

In the next fifty-plus years, Shneidman published twenty books and hundreds of articles on suicide. He wrote the entry for suicide in the *Encyclopædia Britannica*, which he claimed to have read in its entirety when he in high school. Shneidman was one of the founders of the Suicide Prevention Center in Los Angeles, which launched one of the first suicide hotlines in the country in 1962. Two years later he and several others founded the American Association of Suicidology, which today is the preeminent source of research on suicide in the United States.

During a three-year stint as the head of suicide-prevention studies at the National Institute of Mental Health, Shneidman traveled
to forty states sharing his views as a clinician and researcher of the
unbearable psychological pain that leads people to contemplate
suicide. This pain, for which he coined the word *psychache*, was
the key to understanding suicidal behavior, Shneidman maintained. Social statistics and physiological factors have a place, but
suicide is the desperate action of individuals in extreme emotional
duress who can't see other options for relief. Backed into a corner
psychologically, they resort to the one option that is available to
them and offers a guaranteed end to their pain.

Shneidman believed that the only way to explain suicide was to
delve into people's personal history, to learn their individual stories
and glimpse the emotional circumstances behind their desire to die.
In this way, one could begin to make sense of the most perplexing
of all human behaviors.

In 2009 Shneidman died of natural causes at age 91. Up to the
end he said that "no one has to die, absolutely no one. It will be done
for you."[14] He also continued to write, publishing his last book, *A
Commonsense Book of Death*, at age 90.

A Genetic Disposition?

Shneidman had little regard for research that studies physiological
factors, despite evidence that decreased levels of serotonin in the
brain contribute to feelings of depression and thus influence suicidal
behavior. Serotonin, sometimes referred to as one of the "feel-good"
hormones, is a neurotransmitter. Diminished levels of serotonin
have been found in patients who are depressed and have a history of
suicide attempts, as well as in the postmortem brains of suicide victims. (Drugs such as Prozac, Paxil, and Zoloft often are prescribed
to reduce depression because they increase serotonin levels.)

"You don't understand psychopathic murder by slicing [Jeffrey] Dahmer's brain," Shneidman said in a *Los Angeles Times* interview in 2004, "and you won't get $E=MC^2$ by slicing Einstein's brain. Unfortunately, it's in the mind. And the mind is not a structure. It is an ephemeral concept."[15]

That belief is being challenged by current researchers who say that they have found a genetic link to suicide. Scientists at Johns Hopkins University studied 2,700 people with bipolar disorder, 1,200 of whom had attempted suicide and 1,500 who had not. Their findings, which were reported in the *Journal of Molecular Psychiatry*, concluded that a genetic variant in a small region of one chromosome was associated with a greater likelihood of attempted suicide.[16] A similar study in Canada of 3,350 people, 1,200 of whom had a history of suicidal behavior and 2,150 who didn't, also found evidence of a genetic link.[17]

This research is promising in that it may help doctors target one or more genes in the future, although even if it is widely accepted, it won't result in an end-all solution. Having the gene won't mean that an individual is certain to attempt suicide at some point, just as not having it won't guarantee that the person will never attempt suicide. As with most things pertaining to health, and especially suicide, there are exceptions.

Beck and Hopelessness

Aaron T. Beck, a psychiatrist and professor emeritus at the University of Pennsylvania until his death in 2021, viewed the problem somewhat differently. In the 1980s he created the Beck Hopelessness Scale and the Beck Depression Inventory to rate degrees of hopelessness and depression in psychiatric patients as predictors of suicide. In these models, the more one perceives life events as overwhelming, the more despairing he or she becomes. When these events exceed a person's coping abilities and capacity for tolerance, suicidal thoughts and behaviors can develop.

Intuitively that makes sense, although people deal with stressful situations in different ways. Some become hyperanxious, while others are unflustered. Some jump into action, preferring that to sitting and waiting, while others are semiparalyzed. Some are ruled by denial, while for others the focus is on lamenting their fate. The bottom line is that what is unbearable for one person isn't necessarily unbearable for another. Nevertheless, developing effective skills to deal with adversity can mitigate feelings of hopelessness.

Beck studied the records of 207 hospital patients who had been admitted five to ten years earlier because of suicidal ideation, not for a recent attempt. Before learning what had happened to them, he used his hopelessness scale to correctly identify 91 percent of those who had ended up dying by suicide.[18] A subsequent study of 2,000 outpatients yielded similar results, with Beck correctly identifying 94 percent of patients who had eventually killed themselves.[19]

Joiner and Fearlessness

How do people acquire the ability to kill themselves? Wanting to die is one thing; acting on that desire is another. After all, the strongest of all human urges is self-preservation. Voltaire called it "the most powerful instinct of nature."[20] How, one asks, is it possible for some people to voluntarily end their existence before—sometimes a long time before—age or illness do it for them? Is this a sign of weakness, of wanting to escape life, or is it an indication of fearlessness, of being unafraid to die?

It's not unusual for someone who looks down from a great height, whether it's a tall structure or a high mountaintop, to imagine what it would be like to fall. Common sense and good judgment stop most of us from doing anything more than imagining it, though, and if there isn't a solid guardrail, we are careful not to get too close to the edge. In the same way, many individuals who want to die can't bring themselves to jump from the precipice, pull the trigger, swallow poison, cut themselves, or otherwise inflict self-harm. Yet a smaller number of people have this capacity. Moreover, they follow through on it. What makes them different?

Thomas Joiner, the Robert O. Lawton Distinguished Professor of Psychology at Florida State University, is the author of numerous books and studies on suicide. The subject is a professional interest of his and also a personal one because when he was in college his father drove to an office park a mile from home and killed himself in the back of a van.

Joiner believes that the capacity to kill oneself combined with the desire to die is the key to suicide. People not only have to want to die, he says; they have to overcome the natural instinct for self-preservation. How? Through practice and repeated exposure to pain and death. He uses the rock star Kurt Cobain's suicide as an example. As a young man, Cobain was afraid of guns, needles, and heights. At age 27, however, he shot himself after years as a self-injecting drug user who scaled thirty-foot platforms during his concerts. What changed?

Cobain "worked up" to the act of suicide, Joiner says, by acclimating himself to pain and potential danger. The first couple of times that a friend invited him to go shooting, Cobain wouldn't get out of the car. Later, Cobain got out of the car, but he wouldn't touch a gun. Still later, he let his friend teach him how to aim and fire. Through continued exposure, he conquered his fear of guns, and in similar fashion he overcame his aversion to needles and heights.[21]

In much the same way, nonlethal self-injury, such as cutting oneself with a razor blade, a knife, or a piece of glass, and self-induced starvation (anorexia) are gateways to suicide, Joiner believes. Although the intent rarely is lethal, cumulative and escalating experiences prepare a person to be less afraid of dying. Similarly, body piercings, tattoos, and cosmetic surgery can progressively increase one's pain threshold, to the point where even extreme acts, such as dousing oneself with gasoline and setting one's body on fire, no longer seem terrifying.

Past suicide attempts also lead to increased capacity, even if an attempt didn't seem serious to others at the time. Individuals who are, in essence, "trying out" suicide, working through it in their minds in order to decide on a means and perhaps a location, may make some sort of "test run," such as consuming a large but nonlethal dose of medication. This can place them at much greater risk the next time because the danger will seem less threatening. While family members and friends may consider these acts to be calls for attention rather than genuine attempts, they actually contribute to a person's ability to overcome the natural instinct for self-preservation.

"Some people think that those who commit suicide are weak," Joiner says, but "it's actually about fearlessness. You cannot do it unless you are fearless, and this is behavior that is learned."[22] One doesn't have to experience pain and injury personally, however, in order to develop the capacity to kill oneself. Joiner believes that repeated witnessing of pain, violence, or injury is sufficient. This explains why physicians and prostitutes have high suicide rates. Every day they are exposed to pain and suffering, and gradually they become inured to it.

The same is true for police officers and military service members—with an added risk. While physicians have easy access to drugs, cops and troops have easy access to firearms, which are far more deadly. Often this access continues long after they have retired because people in these professions tend to keep guns around them for protection and security.

According to a 2018 study by the Ruderman Family Foundation, police officers witness, on average, 188 "critical incidents" in their career. These traumatic events, in which someone is assaulted, is seriously injured in an accident, suffers a major heart attack or stroke, or is killed, can lead to depression, post-traumatic stress disorder (PTSD), and other forms of mental illness in officers. Because of the shame and stigma associated with asking for help, their symptoms go untreated, leaving them at greater risk for suicide. The study notes that at least 140 police officers killed themselves in 2017. In contrast, 129 police officers died that year in the line of duty. Of the 18,000 law enforcement agencies in the country, only 3–5 percent had suicide-prevention training programs.[23]

Firefighters were included in the study since they also respond to tragedies, and the results for them were similar. In 2017, 103 firefighters died by suicide, compared with 93 who died in the line of duty. The disparity between those who killed themselves and those who died on the job might be even greater for firefighters than for cops, however. The study cites an estimate by the Firefighter Behavioral Health Alliance that as many as 60 percent of firefighter suicides are never reported.[24]

Because police officers and firefighters present a veneer of bravery and toughness, and because their suicides aren't often covered by mainstream media, the public isn't likely to know that these professions have suicide rates that are at least five times that of civilians. An exception occurred in July 2019, when New York City experienced the seventh and eighth suicides by police officers that year. The story received national attention and prompted city officials to refer to the deaths as a "mental health crisis" in need of immediate action. The form that action takes—other than encouraging officers to seek help—remains to be seen, however. Over the previous five years, the NYPD had averaged four or five suicides per year, so this was a definite uptick.

Another exception occurred in the aftermath of the January 6, 2021, insurrection at the White House. In addition to one officer, Brian Sicknick, being killed and more than a thousand rioters being arrested, four members of the Capitol Police who responded to the attack killed themselves later. These four were veterans of eighteen, sixteen, twelve, and five years, respectively. None were newbies. In his testimony before a congressional subcommittee, one Capitol Police officer said, "What we all went through that day was traumatic."[25]

Pairing Capacity with Intent

The capacity to kill oneself isn't enough, however. One must also have the desire, which Joiner says derives either from a perception that one is a burden to others or from a feeling that he or she doesn't belong. Joiner trained a group of people to evaluate real suicide notes in terms of perceived burdensomeness, as well as hopelessness and general emotional pain. What the raters didn't know was that half the notes had been written by people who killed themselves and half had been written by people who survived their suicide attempt. Perceived burdensomeness was more prevalent in the notes of those who had died than in the notes of those who had survived. The former made more lethal attempts because their desire to die was stronger. There was no statistical difference when the notes were evaluated for hopelessness or emotional pain. These findings supported an earlier study in which people who had survived a serious suicide attempt characterized their desire to die as a way to relieve others of the burden of caring for them, while people who had engaged in self-injurious behavior that wasn't suicidal (primarily cutting) characterized their behavior as an expression of anger or a desire to punish themselves.

Referring back to Kurt Cobain's death, Joiner says that the suicide note Cobain left, which was addressed to his wife, implies perceived burdensomeness. "Please keep going," Cobain wrote, "for Frances [their daughter]. Her life will be so much happier without me."[26]

Lack of social connectedness—what Joiner calls "thwarted belongingness"—parallels Durkheim's theory of suicide. In a Norwegian study, one million women were tracked over fifteen years.

The suicide rate of those with six or more children was only one-fifth the rate of other women.[27] A Danish study in 2003 compared 18,000 people who died by suicide with 370,000 others who were randomly selected. It concluded that having children, especially young children, is a buffer against suicide.[28] Another study the same year found that twins have lower rates of suicide regardless of their gender, even though there is evidence suggesting that twins may be slightly more likely to develop mental disorders than non-twins, which in other circumstances would increase the risk of suicide.[29]

"One of the more interesting facets of the possible association between thwarted belongingness and suicide," Joiner says, "is the 'pulling together' effect at times of national tragedy."[30] When it seems as if people should be most depressed because a calamity has befallen the country, in fact they experience a greater sense of social connectedness. The shared experience of a crisis increases an individual's feelings of belonging. It's not surprising that suicide rates in the United States declined during World War I and World War II, then increased immediately afterward. They also declined following the assassination of President John F. Kennedy on November 22, 1963; in fact, a study of twenty-nine major US cities found that there wasn't a single reported suicide for eight days after Kennedy's death, from November 22 to November 30, even though there had been suicides between those dates in the years before, as there would be in the years after.[31] Similar data emerged following the 1986 explosion of the *Challenger* spacecraft and the 9/11 terrorist attacks. Even people who were physically isolated during these events felt socially connected, as if they weren't alone because people all around them were experiencing the same sense of loss. The country was united in its grief, and individual feelings of depression and despair were counterbalanced by the thought that this was normal—it was what everyone else was feeling.

Similarly, suicides rarely occur in concentration camps, where a person's desire to live would seem to be at its lowest point. Despite starvation, cold, torture, and separation from or loss of loved ones, people don't kill themselves. The Italian writer Primo Levi, who survived Auschwitz, wrote in *The Drowned and the Saved,* "The day was dense; one had to think about satisfying hunger, in some way elude fatigue and cold, avoid the blows. Precisely because of the constant imminence of death there was no time to concentrate on the idea of death."[32]

People who return home alive after being imprisoned in a death camp may die by suicide later, however, as Levi did. Only 3 of the 650 prisoners in his original convoy lived to tell about it. Forty-two years later, suffering from severe depression, Levi threw himself down the stairs of his fourth-floor apartment in Turin, "one of numerous death-camp survivors who ultimately took their life," according to George Howe Colt in *November of the Soul.*[33]

Thomas Joiner was able to combine his professional study of suicide with his personal love of sports to prove that the sense of pulling together that results from being a fan provides another form of connectedness. When a city's most popular sports teams, professional or collegiate, win a national championship, there is a temporary decline in the suicide rate. Conversely, after a loss the rate goes up. People literally live and die with their team.

The US men's hockey team's victory over the Soviet Union at the 1980 Winter Olympics—the so-called "Miracle on Ice"—came at a time when the Iran hostage crisis had gone on for 111 days and Russia's invasion of Afghanistan was a month old. Millions of people in America had never seen a hockey game and didn't know the rules or the names of any of the players, yet they were glued to their TV sets and radios rooting the home team to victory. It's not surprising, Joiner says, that the US suicide rate was unusually low that day, February 22, 1980, compared with the same date twenty years before and twenty years after.[34] (It may have been unusually high in the Soviet Union, although no data are available to verify this.)

Joiner's theory of suicide, that people kill themselves because they have both the capacity and the desire to end their lives, can be applied to mass suicides, he maintains. In 1978 Jim Jones induced 914 of his Peoples Temple followers in Guyana to drink grape-flavored Kool-Aid laced with cyanide. In 1997 in Los Angeles, Marshall Applewhite coerced 39 of his Heaven's Gate brethren to ingest a lethal mixture of phenobarbital and vodka. In both instances, prior to the fateful day there were explicit rehearsals for suicide, designed to overcome people's fear of dying. On multiple occasions, Jones tested the loyalty of his followers by giving them a drink that he said contained poison (it didn't) and telling them to swallow it. In Jonestown, people worked long hours in oppressive heat farming and constructing buildings, receiving little food—another way that they became accustomed to suffering. In Heaven's Gate, 8 of the 18 men who died had undergone voluntary castrations.

It's possible to argue that a sense of belongingness exists in cults. After all, people work side by side, eat together, worship together, cohabitate, sometimes share sex partners, and often engage in communal childrearing. Outsiders are demonized, adding to the cult's solidarity, and dissidents are expelled. In fact, though, followers' connection to one another is minimal. Crises are invented to keep the focus on the leader, and close relationships are disrupted so that alternative forms of authority don't develop. As a result, followers don't belong to a group, they belong to the leader, who isn't interested in developing community bonds. His interest (cult leaders almost always are male) is in exerting and maintaining power.

Understanding why people die by suicide is critical to preventing it. At the same time, no two individuals, not even identical twins, are exactly alike. While circumstances may push one person to the brink, causing him or her to consider suicide, the same circumstances might lead others to different choices. It doesn't help that the only person potentially capable of explaining his or her suicidal intentions may not be alive to do so; nevertheless, even people who attempt suicide and survive can't always articulate their motives.

Access to Lethal Means

Examining *how* people die by suicide can be as important as understanding *why* they resort to suicide. It lacks the weight of existential study—Albert Camus referred to suicide as "the one truly serious philosophical problem,"[35] while Shakespeare's Hamlet poses the question that is at the heart of suicide: "To be or not to be." At the same time, a study of methods used in suicides has the benefit of being concrete. While we may never know exactly why a person takes his or her life, we can determine with near 100 percent certainty the method used. Gunshot, poison, hanging, jumping, drowning, stabbing, cutting—each is unmistakable.

Worldwide, the leading method of suicide is hanging. People don't always have access to a gun, drugs, a motor vehicle, or a jump site, but they can fashion a noose out of just about anything. In China, where pesticides are readily available for agricultural purposes, poison is the top choice. In Norway, which is surrounded by water, a disproportionate number of people kill themselves by drowning. In Sri Lanka, the most popular method used to be jumping into a well, until indoor plumbing was introduced and wells became obsolete (now the leading method is pesticide poisoning).[36]

The choice of method rarely is random. Usually it's related to the means that is most available. Police officers invariably shoot themselves because they have access to a firearm. Physicians tend to overdose because they can obtain lethal quantities of drugs easily. Prisoners hang themselves because the only means available to them are bed sheets, shirts, and shoelaces.

In *November of the Soul*, George Howe Colt noted three deaths: one man killed himself by jumping into a vat of beer, a second man locked himself into a high-altitude test chamber, and a third man lay in front of a steamroller. Each was unusual, yet the means were explicable once one learned that the first man was a brewer, the second was an Air Force technician, and the third was a construction worker. They had ready access to the means.

One 47-year-old woman told Colt, "It takes a tremendous amount of energy to figure out how you're going to kill yourself." She considered various options, from jumping off a roof to shooting herself, dismissing each one because death wasn't certain or she didn't want to leave a mess for others to deal with. She ended up parking her car far from her home and inhaling carbon monoxide. When police found her the next morning—unconscious but alive in a sleeping bag, with a vacuum cleaner hose attached to her car's tailpipe—she was rushed to a hospital and revived. Afterward, she said, "I kept thinking about what would be easiest for everyone else. Of course, the easiest thing would have been if I lived."[37]

Anne Sexton also resorted to carbon monoxide, killing herself in 1974 at age 45. Several years before her death she wrote a poem titled "Wanting to Die." It contains these lines: "But suicides have a special language. / Like carpenters they want to know *which tools*. / They never ask *why build*."[38]

The challenge for those who study suicide, as well as for caregivers and family members, is to understand as much as possible about what drives someone to the edge—and beyond. The more we learn, the greater our chances of being able to do something about it.

CHAPTER 3

By the Numbers

MOST EXPERTS BELIEVE THAT SUICIDES ARE UNDERREPORTED— from a little to a lot. It's common for family members to pressure coroners to rule that a loved one's death was the result of an accident rather than suicide because of the stigma of suicide. This is especially true in the case of drug overdoses. If a note isn't found and there isn't strong evidence to the contrary, coroners may comply, or they may at least rule that the manner of death is undetermined. Families also advocate against a ruling of suicide if it would void the decedent's life insurance policy, although any policy that is taken out or renewed more than two years before the person's death can't be nullified.

Another reason why suicides are underreported is that it may be impossible to determine whether a death was in fact accidental. In Arthur Miller's play *Death of a Salesman*, there is no doubt that Willy Loman kills himself by driving into a tree, but other, similar deaths are less obvious. If a car hits an immovable object or goes over an embankment, did the driver fall asleep at the wheel, swerve to avoid an animal, lose control, or intend to die? If the driver had a stroke or a heart attack there will be forensic evidence, but otherwise, in the absence of skid marks or a suicide note, coroners can't tell. Similarly, if someone is found dead in bed as the result of a drug overdose and there isn't a note, was it accidental or intentional?

Despite this dilemma, suicide statistics compiled by the national Centers for Disease Control and Prevention, as well as other resources, are compelling. Suicide is the tenth leading cause of death among adults and the second leading cause among teens (behind accidents), as well as for adults aged 25 to 44 (also behind accidents). Every day now, at least 130 Americans, on average, kill themselves. To put that number in perspective, it's equivalent to 9/11 happening every three and a half weeks. It's also equivalent to a fully loaded commercial airliner crashing every other day.

The psychologist Kay Jamison, in *Night Falls Fast: Understanding Suicide*, published a year before 9/11, notes the magnitude of loss from suicide by comparing it with two prominent events in recent decades, the Vietnam War and the AIDS epidemic. The vast majority of American military victims in Vietnam were males under age 35; even so, there were nearly twice as many suicides of men in this age group who served in the war as there were battlefield deaths (101,732 compared with 54,708, according to Jamison). Males under 35 also made up the largest number of AIDS victims, yet 15,000 more young men died by suicide during the height of the epidemic than from AIDS.[1]

Adult Suicides

There are two ways to measure suicide—by the total number of deaths and by the number of deaths per 100,000 people. The latter method takes into account changes in population size, enabling comparisons between years, regional areas, and various demographic groups. It is determined by multiplying the number of suicides in a targeted population by 100,000, then dividing by the population size. Thus, one suicide among 10,000 people equals a suicide rate of 10. One suicide in a school of 2,000 students equals a suicide rate of 50. In 1981 the national rate was 12.0. Since then it has vacillated from a low of 10.5 in 1999 to 14.5 today.[2]

Historically, seniors in America have always had the highest suicide rates. One reason is that they tend to be more socially isolated, often living alone. Once they are retired they no longer have daily interaction with coworkers and may not feel useful anymore. They also may face financial hardships or believe that they are a burden to others. On top of this, while young people often are depressed by problems that are for the most part transitory, elderly people face problems that are more likely to be permanent, such as loss of partners, friends, mobility, career, vision, hearing, and good health. Unlike younger people, seniors are more often driven to suicide by a sense of loneliness than by anger or drug abuse. As a result, seniors tend to be more deliberate in their planning, less ambivalent about their intentions, and less interested in leaving the outcome to chance.

Yet there is a paradox.

"For people ages 20 to 34, suicide is the second leading cause of death," says Stephen Dubner, the host of *Freakonomics*, "and it's in the top five for all Americans from ages 15 to 54." Yet among seniors "suicide isn't even a top-ten cause of death," he notes. This is because people who are elderly die from many things—heart disease, cancer, accidental falls—so suicide is farther down the list.[3]

In recent years, suicide rates among adults aged 45 to 64 have risen sharply, at times overtaking the rates of senior suicides.[4] "This is concerning," says Kate Scannell, a physician and syndicated columnist, "because we expect and hope to see these people at the high point of their lives, enjoying what they've accomplished and the lives they've built, sailing the robust current of the great American dream into their secure future."[5] A number of theories attempt to explain the rise, including the increased use and abuse of opiates, as well as the mortgage crisis that started in 2008 and continues to be felt by many people today.[6]

A study published in the *Journal of Public Health* noted that suicides doubled between 2005 and 2010, when home evictions and foreclosures were at their highest.[7] Even more important, though, is that a growing number of jobs are being automated, phased out, or moved overseas. Since the decade before retirement is when the earnings of most workers are at their peak, adding to their nest egg for the future, people in this age group feel the effect of corporate cutbacks, layoffs, and downsizing more than others.

According to a study by the CDC, the suicide rate in 1928—the earliest year for which data are available—was 18 per 100,000 adults. By 1932, the last full year of the Depression, it had climbed to 22.1. This represented a 23 percent jump over four years, the largest increase in American history prior to 2020 and the coronavirus pandemic. Between 1932 and 2007, according to the study, the overall suicide rate dropped to 11.2; however, there were smaller increases in 1937–38 (the end of Franklin D. Roosevelt's New Deal), in 1973–75 (when the oil crisis was at its height), and in 1980–82 (when the country was in a recession), each tied to the economy.[8]

In terms of occupation, some have a higher risk of suicide than others. Another CDC report, based on a study of 12,312 deaths in seventeen states, found that three occupational groups were particularly at risk of suicide. One group was people in farming, fishing, and forestry, whose suicide rate—84.5—was nearly six times the national rate. The second was people in construction and extraction (i.e., mining and fossil fuels), whose rate of 53.3 was three and a half times the national rate. The third group was people in installation, maintenance, and repair, at 47.9. What the three groups had in common was work that tended to be seasonal and to be performed by males.

The occupations with the lowest suicide rate—7.5—were in education, training, and library services. Workers in these professions, the report noted, are predominantly female and may not be their family's primary breadwinner, so that there is less stress on the family if the job is lost. The highest rate of suicide among females—14—was, no surprise, in protective services, primarily law enforcement and firefighting.[9]

An interesting side note regarding the connection between employment and suicide is that according to a 2019 study in the *American Journal of Preventive Medicine*, states that have increased their minimum wage have lower suicide rates. Researchers examined data on minimum wages and suicide rates in all fifty states over ten years, from 2006 to 2016, and found that every dollar increase in a state's minimum wage was associated with a 1.9 percent decrease in its annual suicide rate.[10]

Said Alex Gartner, of the University of North Carolina at Chapel Hill, who led the study, "It's possible that increasing the minimum wage improves life satisfaction, increases access to health care, and decreases mental illness, which all lead to fewer suicide deaths. . . . We can't say for sure that slower growth in suicide rates is caused by increasing minimum wages, but it warrants further study."[11] He didn't add—but the report did—that an annual decrease of 1.9 percent in the suicide rate during the study period equaled eight thousand fewer deaths.

In the midst of Covid-19, many young adults, in particular, reported suicidal thoughts. According to the CDC, a survey of more than five thousand adults from June 24 to June 30, 2020 revealed that one in four people aged 18 to 24 had seriously considered suicide in the previous thirty days.[12] No one was immune to the stress of the pandemic, but for those who were trying to finish college or find a job or sustain friendships while being socially isolated, it was especially challenging. It was even more challenging for health care workers, first responders, and everyone in service industries—from supermarket checkers to gas station attendants, teachers to garbage collectors—particularly parents in these professions who had young or teenage children at home. Worse, Covid-19 wasn't limited to a specific time and place as 9/11 or natural disasters were. It was everywhere, with every country having to deal with it.

My local newspaper, the *San Francisco Chronicle*, reported in August 2020 that calls to San Francisco Suicide Prevention from individuals who were considered to be at medium to high risk of suicide had increased by 25 percent during the early months of the coronavirus and were continuing to increase each month thereafter. Across the bay, Crisis Support Services of Alameda County, whose service area includes Oakland and Berkeley, reported that calls from people at medium to high risk of suicide had increased by 272 percent since the start of the pandemic.[13] Anxiety and depression were mounting, owing partly to shelter-in-place requirements, partly to a record number of job losses and the ensuing economic uncertainty, and partly to the rapidly growing number of people who had died from the virus. Among those hardest hit have been African Americans, Latinos, and the elderly, but no segment of the population has been spared, meaning that in many instances people haven't been able to rely on family members or friends for help. They have had to face the "new normal" alone.

Youth Suicides

Every suicide is tragic, but in many respects suicides among young people are the most tragic of all. They had so much of their life still ahead of them, we think, with all the promise that it held. For it to be cut short by their own hand is hard to fathom. If only, we wish, they could have held on a little longer and gotten the help they needed, everything would have been different. A young person's suicide throws off the whole order of life and gives everyone who knows about it reason to pause. The Japanese have a saying: "White hair should go before black hair," meaning that old people should die before young people.

In 2020 more than five hundred children aged 10 to 14 killed themselves, according to the CDC, making suicide the second leading cause of death in that group, behind unintentional injury. Among young adults aged 15 to 24 the number of suicide deaths in 2020 was roughly six thousand, making it the number-two cause of death in that age group as well.[14]

Youths who attempt suicide often are influenced by factors that are mystic, romantic, or idealistic in nature. In addition, their actions, much more than those of adults, are motivated by anger, risk-taking, and drug abuse. Another factor is that youths from middle- and upper-income families tend to have high expectations placed on them by parents who are successful professionally. They are pushed to excel in school, be popular among peers, develop a talent in music, drama, art, or sports, and participate in extracurricular activities not because they enjoy them but because it looks good on a college application. When they fail a test or suffer a romantic breakup, the result can be devastating, especially if they haven't had to deal with failure before. In contrast, low-income kids usually face adversity growing up—frequent moves, potential homelessness, periodic hunger—and develop coping skills as a result.

According to a psychologist quoted in George Howe Colt's book *November of the Soul,* "One of the most important things we can do for our children is build some failure into their lives so they learn that it is possible to fail without being a failure." Jerry Motto, a San Francisco psychiatrist, went further. "Early on," he said, "we should give children puzzles they can't solve—and then give them love when they fail."[15]

Other Factors

Among the strongest risk factors for suicides in adolescents is childhood trauma, particularly abuse. Two researchers who reviewed twenty studies determined that adults who had been sexually or physically abused as children were up to twenty-five times as likely to attempt suicide as adults who had not been. The longer the period of abuse and the closer the relationship of the abuser to the victim, the greater the risk of suicide. Childhood abuse often leads to low self-esteem, substance abuse, delinquent behavior, and detachment from others—all tied to suicide risk.[16]

Alcohol is its own risk factor. As a depressant, it makes someone who already is depressed even more so, while decreasing inhibitions and providing "liquid courage" to act on plans that are poorly thought out. "Autopsies tell us that one-third to one-half of teenage suicides are under the influence of alcohol or drugs shortly before they kill themselves," writes George Howe Colt, "while nearly one-third of teenage attempters are drunk or high shortly before they attempt."[17] Combined with access to a firearm, alcohol can be deadly. According to a study in the *Journal of the American Medical Association*, teenagers who use a gun in a suicide attempt are five times more likely to have been drinking than those who resort to other means of suicide.[18]

Then there is bullying. Yesterday's bullies were physically intimidating, but that was all. Almost exclusively male, they called other boys names and made threats, sometimes stole another student's lunch money or damaged property, but only infrequently hit or kicked. Today's bullies are different. The more subtle ones, especially females, humiliate and manipulate, isolate and ostracize. The most worrisome, usually males, resort to violence, everything from punching or stabbing their victims to burning or shooting them.

Yesterday's victims dealt with bullies largely by avoiding them. The thinking was that after a time bullies would get bored and find another target. Today's victims, like today's bullies, are different. In the most extreme cases, victims fight back with firepower, killing their tormentors and often themselves, ending a murder spree with their suicide. According to the National Threat Assessment Center, in more than two-thirds of all school shootings the attacker felt persecuted, bullied, or threatened. Bullied students also are more than twice as likely as their non-bullied peers to bring guns or knives to school.[19] According to the US Department of Education, 21 percent of students reported being bullied at school.[20]

The latest form of bullying is cyberbullying, in which cell phones and computers are used to spread harmful rumors and send hurtful texts, as well as to post mean comments, fake profiles, and embarrassing pictures and videos on social media sites. Cyberbullying is even more insidious in many respects than physical bullying because it can happen anytime, day or night, often when the victim is alone. In addition, comments and images can be posted anonymously and distributed rapidly to a large number of people. This makes it difficult for anyone to identify the source or to delete inappropriate and harassing texts and pictures after they have been posted or sent. The shame and embarrassment a victim feels when he or she is physically bullied are magnified when the bullying takes the form of cyberbullying because it seems as if everyone knows about it.

A 2015 survey by the CDC found that 15 percent of high school students had been victims of cyberbullying in the previous twelve months.[21] One reason that suicide rates for girls have been increasing in recent years, especially in girls aged 10 to 14, is that girls are more vulnerable to the effects of social media. "Compared with boys, girls use social media more frequently and are more likely to experience cyberbullying," according to a 2019 study published in *JAMA*.[22]

Cultural assimilation issues can be a source of stress for youths whose parents grew up in another country, while they were born in the United States and have lived their whole lives here. Parents don't understand why their children want to wear certain clothes, have certain hairstyles, or get piercings and tattoos. If parents prohibit them and they obey, the youths may end up ostracized at school. If they rebel in order to conform with peers, however, it creates conflict at home.

If a teen is feeling suicidal and confides in anyone, most likely it's a close friend, who is made to promise not to tell anyone. Among suicide-prevention advocates this is referred to as "the deadly secret." It becomes an enormous burden for anyone, especially a young person, to bear. The close friend doesn't want his or her friend to get hurt but also doesn't want to betray the friend's confidences. What to do?

The answer, as difficult as it may be, is for the friend asked to keep the secret to tell a trusted adult—a teacher, counselor, coach, or parent. What might seem like an act of betrayal can be the gift of a lifetime. Then it's the responsibility of the adult to act, following protocols and procedures that are set by the school or in consultation with a mental health provider who is experienced in suicide prevention.

Gender Differences

On average, there are more than 130 suicides every day in America, or one every eleven minutes. Seventy percent of them are by males. Among men, the age group with the highest rate—38.8 per 100,000—is 75 and older. Among women, the suicide rate is highest for those 45 to 64 (9.8 per 100,000).

There isn't a complete count of suicide attempts, mainly because many attempts don't result in hospitalization and aren't reported to anyone. The CDC gathers data from hospitals regarding nonfatal injuries from self-harm, however, so a few things are known. By comparing the number of people who are hospitalized in a given year following a suicide attempt with the number of people who kill themselves that same year, it's possible to estimate that for every reported death by suicide twelve people harm themselves. In addition, the ratio of attempts to suicides among youths is estimated to be as high as 100 to 1, while for the elderly, whose attempts tend to be more determined and more lethal, the ratio is 4 to 1.[23]

Although males are three times as likely to die by suicide as females, females make three to four times as many attempts. The reason for this disparity is that most males use a firearm, while most females overdose. A gunshot wound to the head is almost always fatal, while the effects of swallowing a bottle of pills can be reversed if others act quickly.

In 2017 the CDC released the results of a study in which researchers analyzed data from the years 2001 to 2015 on nonfatal, self-inflicted injuries that resulted in emergency room treatment. The study included fourteen thousand boys and twenty-nine thousand girls aged 10 to 24. The sharpest increase occurred among the youngest girls, aged 10 to 14, whose rate tripled to 318 hospital visits per 100,000, while the highest rate—633 visits per 100,000—was among older teen girls. The rate for young women aged 20 to 24 increased as well but at a slower pace, from 228 visits in 2001 to 346 in 2015. Somewhat surprisingly, rates for boys didn't change much, researchers noted.[24]

Researchers at Vanderbilt University reached the same conclusion. They studied children and teens treated for suicidal thoughts and behaviors at forty-nine major US children's hospitals in the years 2008 to 2015. Two-thirds were girls, and the number of visits during that seven-year span nearly doubled. Half the visits were by older teens, but among those aged 12 to 14 there was a 37 percent increase. Also of note, the rate of hospitalization was considerably higher during the school year, indicating that academic stresses and social pressures played a significant part.[25]

Related to social pressure is another disparity between genders when it comes to youth suicide. It has to do with how boys and girls react to a peer's suicide attempt if that attempt becomes public knowledge. Boys who attempt suicide and survive often experience increased ridicule from other boys. "He's such a loser, he couldn't even kill himself," they say, as if killing oneself were easy but the victim couldn't manage it. As a result, the poor boy is shunned even more and tends to withdraw further from others, until he is primarily or exclusively alone. This puts him at greater risk for another suicide attempt, sometimes after he plots—and in some instances carries out—revenge against his tormentors first.

For girls, the reaction to a suicide attempt can be quite different. Rather than feeling a diminished sense of worth, some girls experience elevated social standing. "She was feeling so bad that she actually tried to kill herself," other girls say with awe and even a sense of envy, as if they have never descended to such depths but can empathize with someone who has. Whereas boys may experience increased scorn from peers following an attempt, girls may experience increased esteem.

According to a 2011 CDC report, 30 percent of high school girls had seriously considered suicide during the previous twelve months, 24 percent had made a plan, 13 percent had made an attempt, and 4 percent had required medical care related to their attempt. The numbers for boys were roughly half those for girls: 14 percent had seriously considered suicide, 12 percent had made a plan, 7 percent had made an attempt, and 2 percent had required medical treatment for an attempt. Moreover, 60 percent of high school girls said that they felt sad or hopeless, double the percentage for boys and the highest percentage in a decade.[26]

Ethnic Differences

Native Americans and Alaska natives have the highest suicide rate in the United States (22.2 per 100,000 in 2017), followed by whites (17.8), Hispanics (6.9), African Americans (6.9), and Asian/Pacific Islanders (6.8).[27]

"If you're white and in psychological pain, what can you blame it on?" asks the suicide researcher David Lester. "Other people are doing well; why aren't you? Maybe that, in part, accounts for the higher suicide rate in whites compared to African Americans, because whites have fewer external causes to blame for their misery."[28] Another possible reason is that African Americans tend to be more spiritually oriented than whites, and religious taboos discourage behavior that the church doesn't condone. Elderly Black women, in particular, have an unusually low rate of suicide—roughly 2 per 100,000.[29] This is attributed to a strong matriarchal tradition in which Black grandmothers often play a significant role within a family, caring for children, preparing meals, and often keeping house. As a result, they have more say in the way things are run than many white grandmothers.

George Howe Colt suggests a different way of looking at it. He says that elderly Black men and women have had to make "a certain peace with their lives in a racist society, scaling down their hopes to fit reality more closely."[30]

According to a study in the journal *Pediatrics*, suicide attempts by Black high school students increased by 73 percent from 1991 to 2017. Many of the risk factors for suicide—depression, trauma, a parent's death—were amplified in Black families by high poverty rates, disproportionate exposure to violence, and reduced access to medical care owing to lack of insurance and/or lack of transportation.[31]

The coronavirus has heightened the disparity, as has the national reckoning with racism after the killing of unarmed Blacks like George Floyd, Breonna Taylor, and others by white police officers. Black people have died from Covid-19 at higher rates than whites, and like all survivors they have had to grieve in isolation, without funerals and memorial services.

In August 2020, at the height of the pandemic, the CDC reported that 11 percent of all adults had seriously considered suicide in the previous thirty days. Among individuals who identified as either African American or Hispanic, however, the numbers were even higher, 15 percent for Blacks and 19 percent for Hispanics.[32] That said, it's surprising in many respects that the rate of Black suicide wasn't higher. For one thing, Blacks typically underutilize mental health services for financial reasons (lack of health insurance), historical reasons (skepticism of treatment that in the past was substandard), and cultural reasons (e.g., the belief that depression is a "personal weakness" that is better treated with prayer than with prescribed medication). Nevertheless, the connection between depression, mental illness, and suicide is lower for Blacks than for whites.

At this point it's worth repeating something I learned while studying Civil War suicides for my book *The Last and Greatest Battle*. Prior to the war, most whites considered suicide to be a sin, while Blacks generally accepted it. After the war, these attitudes flipped. White society needed a way to explain the startling number of suicides that occurred after the war, especially among people of social standing. Many wealthy farmers and businessmen, especially in the South, who lost their fortunes in the war and their slaves afterward subsequently killed themselves. When this happened, the attitude of white society began to shift. The deaths weren't condoned, but nor were they denounced. Instead of calling suicide a "horrid affair" or a "terrible deed," as they had in the past, news accounts focused on a person's life rather than on his or her death. Negative judgments were replaced by expressions of condolence, sadness, and lament.[33]

For Blacks it was the opposite. In the antebellum South, slaves who died by suicide often were viewed as martyrs. A permissiveness existed because suicide was seen as an acceptable response to human bondage. Moreover, it had elements of rebelliousness in it. By killing themselves, slaves were resisting the authority of their owners and exerting their autonomy in the only way available to them. Black newspapers often applauded their defiance.[34]

It wasn't lost on the Black community that slave owners suffered in multiple ways when a slave resorted to suicide. The money that the owner had invested in purchasing and maintaining the slave was forfeited, owners lost an important asset—the slave's labor—and the reputation of owners took a hit because a slave's suicide implied an owner's cruelty. This isn't to say that suicides among slaves were commonplace before the war or to suggest that they were celebrated. Rather, suicide was viewed as a last resort in the face of extreme stress.[35]

After the war, however, many Blacks believed that the end of slavery opened new doors for them. With emancipation, Blacks had bona fide opportunities for personal advancement, or so they believed. Even though resentful whites blocked efforts by Blacks to gain full citizenship and benefit from economic equality during Reconstruction and later, a sense of optimism existed among Blacks. This optimism united Black communities and meant that suicides ceased to generate the same level of sympathy after the war as they had before it.[36]

As for Native Americans, their suicides rates are among the highest in the United States, twice the rate of the country as a whole and even higher among youths.[37] For adult Native Americans, losing their land; being confined to reservations, where they no longer can support their families; and having to depend on welfare have led to a huge loss of self-esteem, which in turn has resulted in high rates of alcoholism and drug abuse. One study of Cheyenne Indians noted that they were forbidden to hold ritualistic dances and other cultural celebrations and that the men were forced by a government health program to cut their long hair, which was an important symbol of strength.[38]

The Inuit of Alaska, Canada, and Greenland also have high suicide rates—80 per 100,000. One survey found that a third of Inuit youths in a small Arctic community had attempted suicide within the previous six months.[39] The problem among the Inuit is partly economic: subsistence hunting and fishing have diminished over time. In addition, many elderly Inuit walk away quietly to die so that the tribe's resources are preserved. Suicide also is prevalent among

Inuit youths, however, whose prospects for a happy life are dim. Some Inuit youths are separated from their families through forced attendance at distant boarding schools, while nearly all face limited opportunities for employment, live in poor housing, have inadequate sanitation, and miss out on cultural traditions. (For an excellent and entertaining movie that addresses the prevalence of suicides among Inuit youths, see *The Grizzlies*, produced in 2018 and based on a true story. It's about a small town in the Artic where Inuit students are introduced to lacrosse, a sport that initially mystifies them and eventually becomes their passion, lifting them out of depression.)[40]

Geographic Differences

The states with the highest suicide rates are in the West—Nevada, Alaska, Idaho, Arizona, and New Mexico. In terms of actual numbers, California has more suicides than anywhere else in the country—about four thousand suicides per year, or nearly 12 percent of the national total—but California is also the most populous state. The suicide rate in California is the fifth lowest in the country.

There are several reasons why western states have high suicide rates relative to the rest of the United States. Some people go west to find themselves, in the process experiencing geographic dislocation and greater isolation from family members and other support systems. For many, the West may start out representing hope and a fresh beginning—the pot of gold at the end of the rainbow, the chance to begin life anew without the past hanging over them—but over time it can become the end of the trail.

Western states, in particular Alaska and Idaho, have a high proportion of men, especially white men, who are more prone than white women or men or women of color to suicide. Moreover, they tend to adhere strongly to a rugged sense of independence and self-reliance, dating back to frontier days, and are less likely to reach out for help. Arizona and New Mexico, meanwhile, have a high proportion of senior citizens, and the risk of suicide among seniors is pronounced. Florida is the one eastern state with a high percentage of elderly residents; not coincidentally it has a higher than average suicide rate. As for Nevada, its place at the top of the list isn't surprising. The state is a magnet for transient, divorced, and socially withdrawn people. Many of them hope to reverse their fortunes and instead end up gambling away what little they have, adding to their depression and despair.

Another factor is whether people reside in a rural or an urban area. People in rural areas generally have less access to mental health services and emergency care and are more likely to be uninsured. "People who don't have insurance likely can't afford to seek out the kind of help they need, or they may not even know where to look for help, especially in rural areas," says Danielle Steelesmith, coauthor of a 2019 study in the journal *JAMA Network Open* on suicide rates by county. According to the study, which analyzed more than 450,000 suicides from 1996 to 2016, rural areas have a suicide rate that is 25 percent higher than the rate in large cities. Individuals counties with high rates of suicide include those in Appalachian states (Kentucky, Virginia, and West Virginia) as well as less populated counties in Missouri and Arkansas.[41]

States and counties with high rates of suicide have in common a high rate of gun ownership and liberal gun laws. According to the same *JAMA* report, five of the states with the highest suicide rates— Montana (29.6 suicides per 100,000 residents), Wyoming (27.1), Alaska (27.0), New Mexico (23.5), and Idaho (22.8)—have weak gun laws, making access to firearms easy. Conversely, the five states with the lowest suicide rates—New York (8.5), New Jersey (8.8), Massachusetts (9.9), Maryland (10.4), and California (10.9)—have strong gun laws and low rates of gun ownership.[42] A study in the *American Journal of Psychiatry* reached the same conclusion. States with the toughest gun control laws have the lowest suicide rates, researchers said, while the ten states with the weakest gun control laws have suicide rates that are more than twice as high.[43]

The *JAMA Network Open* study notes one exception to the rule that urban areas have lower suicide rates than rural areas. Neighborhoods with gun shops have higher rates of suicide than surrounding neighborhoods. "This is a new variable that hasn't really been looked at," says Steelesmith, "so that definitely needs more research, but we think it is about accessibility."[44] According to one researcher, "Places with fewer gun shops may be places where guns are harder to buy, or they may be places where the local population is more averse to owning guns, or they may be places where local ordinances put limits on gun ownership."[45]

Sexual Orientation and Suicide

It's difficult to quantify the extent of suicide among gays and lesbians. Death records don't include a person's sexual orientation, and it might not be referenced in a suicide note. A similar problem exists when it comes to quantifying suicide attempts, although in 2016 the US Department of Health and Human Services reported that gay and lesbian youths were four times as likely to attempt suicide as heterosexual youths, and their attempts were four to six times as likely to result in an injury that required medical treatment.[46]

A 2020 study by the Trevor Project, a large, crisis-intervention and suicide-prevention service for LGBTQ youths, drew a similar conclusion. Among thirty-five thousand lesbian, gay, bisexual, transgender, and questioning youths aged 13 to 24, more than 40 percent had "seriously considered attempting suicide in the past year." In addition, the LGBTQ respondents who had actually attempted suicide comprised 31 percent of Native/Indigenous respondents, 21 percent of Black and multiracial respondents,

19 percent of whites, 18 percent of Latinx, and 12 percent of Asian/ Pacific Islanders.[47]

It's important to note that the higher rate of suicide attempts among gay and lesbian youths is owing not to their feelings about their sexual orientation but rather to negative reaction to it. Gay and lesbian youths are much more likely to face rejection, isolation, verbal harassment, and physical violence than heterosexual youths. In addition, often they lack the social supports that are available to straight youth. A survey of 3,365 students in Massachusetts in 1995 found that gay and lesbian youths whose families rejected them because of their sexual orientation were more than eight times as likely to attempt suicide as LGBTQ youths whose families were accepting.[48]

Multiple studies have found that gay and lesbian youths have higher rates of depression and anxiety disorders than heterosexual youths, as well as higher rates of alcohol and drug abuse. The former are caused in large part by the stress of being marginalized by society, while the latter are a consequence of a social life in which bars are among the few accepted gathering places. One study found that among male twins where one twin was gay and the other wasn't, the gay twin was twice as likely to consider suicide and nearly four times as likely to attempt it.[49] Another study, of nearly a thousand gays and lesbians in the San Francisco Bay Area, found that 20 percent had attempted suicide before the age of 20.[50]

In a similar vein, a Columbia University psychologist and researcher studied thirty-two thousand eleventh-grade students in Oregon from 2006 to 2008. She created a social index that rated counties in the state on the basis of prevalence of same-sex couples, registered Democratic voters, schools with gay-straight alliances, and schools with anti-bullying and antidiscrimination policies that included sexual orientation. Overall, 25 percent of gay teens in low-scoring counties attempted suicide, compared with 20 percent in high-scoring counties. Among straight teens, the difference was even greater, with 9 percent more attempted suicides in low-scoring communities than in high-scoring ones.[51]

Statistics on transgender individuals are even harder to come by. If they sought medical treatment such as sex reassignment surgery or hormone therapy, some information exists; however, this represents only a subgroup of the transgender population. One study in Sweden determined that people who underwent sex reassignment surgery were nineteen times as likely to die by suicide as people in the general population.[52] That finding has been used to argue against having the procedure; however, it's a questionable comparison because trans people, whether they have had the surgery or not, face the same kinds of rejection, discrimination, harassment, and violence as gays. A different and in many respects more relevant study found that 40 percent of transgender people had made a suicide attempt, 92 percent of them before age 25.[53]

Avoiding Generalizations

At this point a person might be tempted to suggest that the model suicide victim—if one wants to call it that—is an older, white, rural-dwelling, gun-owning, gay male who lives alone. This isn't necessarily wrong, but it implies that anyone who is younger, is a person of color, lives in a city, is female, doesn't own a gun, is heterosexual, and cohabitates is at lesser risk. Each factor—age, culture, race, geography, gun ownership, gender, sexual orientation, and living situation—carries its own set of risks, and there isn't strong empirical evidence that proves one has more or less weight than another. Add mental illness, family history, and substance abuse to the mix, and it becomes even more difficult to make generalizations.

The only conclusion we can make with confidence is that suicide doesn't discriminate on the basis of demographics. Young or old, rich or poor, Black or white, religious or agnostic—it doesn't matter. No group is exempt.

Sports and Suicide

The list in chapter 1 of famous people who have killed themselves includes a number of athletes. One reason is that people who have enjoyed adulation and success throughout their young lives sometimes have a hard time adjusting when their playing days end. The roar of the crowd is gone, the adrenaline rush that accompanies top-level competition no longer is there, big paychecks most likely have ceased, locker-room camaraderie is absent, and trainers and agents aren't around to provide round-the-clock personal care. Most athletes who leave the game are still young by professional standards, but whereas others in their thirties have begun to establish themselves in a long-term career, athletes are just starting out and may not be prepared for life after sports.

Another reason is that many athletes leave the game with a beat-up body. They were in peak physical shape when they first started playing, but overuse of joints and muscles and also injuries have taken a mental as well as a physical toll. It's hard to say good-bye to the limelight and sometimes even harder to adjust to life afterward—chronic pain, decreased mobility, and possibly, if they have suffered concussions, permanent brain impairment.

In recent years, the results of studies on CTE—chronic traumatic encephalopathy, or degeneration caused by repeated head trauma—have raised troubling concerns. At this time there isn't an accurate diagnostic test for CTE in living brains—it only can be found after death, during autopsies—but if that changes, it "will be a moment of reckoning," says Chris Nowinski, a behavioral bioscientist who played football in college. He notes that 99 percent of former NFL players whose brains have been examined posthumously had CTE, and more than a few died by suicide, including the one-time All-Pro linebacker Junior Seau, who killed himself in 2012. His death was the twelfth suicide of a NFL player in twenty-five years. "There's a known and incredibly strong relationship between concussions and increased risk of suicide," Nowinski says. "Most studies suggest a three to four times greater risk from just one concussion."[54]

It's not just football players who are at risk of suicide. Early in 2023 the horseracing world was stunned by the suicides of two jockeys. One of them was a friend of Mike Smith, who won the Triple Crown in 2018 at the age of 52, is still riding, and is in the Racing Hall of Fame. Smith has known other riders who killed themselves. "This is not all of a sudden just happening," he said. "It's been going on. You just never heard of it."[55]

Horseracing presents its own challenges. First and most obviously, it's extremely dangerous. According to the president and CEO of the Jockeys' Guild, each year two jockeys, on average, die from racing, and sixty others are paralyzed. The concussions that jockeys get from falling off a horse at high speed are as violent as the collisions of football players, and jockeys wear less protective gear. Add to this the challenge of maintaining a low weight, which results in eating disorders, plus frequent criticism from owners, trainers, and bettors, and it's not surprising that jockeys suffer a variety of mental health issues. A 2021 report based on interviews with eighty-four jockeys in Ireland found that 80 percent of them had at least one diagnosable mental disorder, with 35 percent suffering from depression and 61 percent meeting the threshold for alcohol abuse.[56]

Female athletes are at risk too. According to a 2017 study by the American Academy of Orthopedic Surgeons, in sports where both boys and girls compete, albeit separately, girls are 12 percent more likely to suffer a concussion than boys. In girls' soccer, for instance, concussions constitute 27 percent of all injuries, possibly because heading the ball is common in soccer.[57]

To date, only one female athlete has been diagnosed with CTE—a former Australian rules football player named Heather Anderson. She played seven games in 2017, retired later that year, and killed herself in 2022 at age 28. Her family donated her brain to the Australian Sports Brain Bank, and the director there reported that he found "multiple CTE lesions as well as abnormalities nearly everywhere I looked in her cortex."[58] In the United States, two former World Cup stars, Brandi Chastain and Michelle Akers, have expressed public concern over memory-loss issues and said that they will participate in a CTE study at Boston University. It remains to be seen whether CTE in female athletes results in an increased suicide risk, but if the experience of football players is any indication, it's a strong possibility.

Then there is baseball. In 1989, shortly before former All-Star pitcher Donnie Moore shot himself after shooting his wife (she survived; he didn't), a researcher at the University of Southern Maine recommended that Major League Baseball players receive counseling after they retire. His reason was that seventy-seven former MLB players had killed themselves. More than half were in their late twenties to late forties,[59] when they most felt their absence from the game and their future plans were uncertain.

Players and former players aren't the only people at risk of suicide, however. Their fans are too. In chapter 2 I referenced Thomas Joiner's study regarding the decrease in suicides immediately following the US hockey team's "Miracle on Ice" Olympic victory in 1980. Joiner has conducted other studies that show a link between the success or failure of a sports team and suicide. For example, he found that fewer suicides occur in America on the Sunday when the Super Bowl is played than on other Sundays during the year. Also, he determined that there is a correlation between the national rankings of the football teams at Florida State University, where Joiner is a tenured professor, and Ohio State University, which is a perennial football powerhouse, and suicides in the cities where the universities are located. When the teams were highly ranked, the suicide rates in Gainesville, Florida, and Columbus, Ohio, were lower, Joiner found.[60]

Other studies support this finding. In one study of thirty metropolitan areas in the United States over twenty years, the suicide rate went down when the area's pro team made the playoffs and went on to win a championship.[61] In another study, the defeat of a high-profile soccer team in England led to an increase in cases of self-poisoning.[62] In a third study, suicides of young men increased in Quebec when the Montreal Canadians hockey team lost an early-round playoff series.[63]

People joke sometimes about "living and dying" with their favorite team, but the sense of belongingness that a person feels in rooting for a team can be undone when that team loses and its season is over. It's easy to say that no one should take sports so seriously, but as a fan myself, I'm aware of the lure.

Popular Times of Suicide

Research in the 1960s cited by David Lester reveals that most suicides occur between noon and 6:00 p.m., with far fewer suicides between midnight and 6:00 a.m.[64] George Howe Colt agrees with the latter. "Though it is commonly assumed that most suicides take place in the dark recesses of the night," he says, "they are more likely to occur in the morning, which may constitute a sort of miniature version of spring: The world is getting up and starting anew—why can't I?"[65] Recent research contradicts this view, however. According to a 2018 study, there are more suicides between midnight and 4:00 a.m. than at any other time. "Not only are nightmares and insomnia significant risk factors for suicidal ideation," said the report's main author, "but just being awake at night may in and of itself be a risk factor."[66]

Although more research needs to be done to determine whether either conclusion is valid, there is general agreement when it comes to the day of the week and the months of the year that are most popular. The day is Monday, and the peak months are April and May.

Mondays are popular because they represent the start of the work week for most adults and the start of the school week for most students. Any relief that the weekend provided—from the grind of a job, annoying coworkers, or the torment of classmates—is over. People are thrust back into the maelstrom. The depression that sets in on Mondays is reflected in the lyrics of popular songs: "It's just another manic Monday; I wish it was Sunday," "Rainy days and Mondays always get me down," "Every other day of the week is fine, yeah, but whenever Monday comes you can find me cryin' all of the time." The least popular day for suicide—no surprise—is Saturday.

As far as the calendar goes, it's logical to think that most suicides occur in winter. On the first page of *Moby Dick*, Herman Melville described Ishmael's suicidal depression as "a damp, drizzly November of my soul," hence the title of Colt's book, *November of the Soul*. Add to this the hustle and bustle of the holidays, when some people feel left out, or the dread of getting together with family members whom a person might prefer to avoid, and the days leading up to a major holiday like Thanksgiving or Christmas would seem to be peak suicide times. In fact, however, suicide rates are highest in the spring. It's a time of rebirth, but not for everyone.

T. S. Eliot's poem "The Waste Land" starts with these oft-repeated words: "April is the cruelest month." It goes on to say that "winter kept us warm, covering Earth in forgetful snow," but the new life evoked by spring is temporary, and hope that ends up being unfulfilled leads to the worst sort of pain. Susanna Kaysen said the same thing in a different way. In her memoir *Girl, Interrupted*, subsequently made into a movie, she wrote about the eighteen months she spent in a psychiatric hospital. At one point she notes, "It was a spring day, the sort that gives people hope: all soft winds and delicate smells of warm earth. Suicide weather."[67]

Depression may start in winter, but it's most intense in spring. Just as people are united by a large-scale disaster that doesn't affect them personally but affects them mentally, producing gloom but also a sense of togetherness, so too are people affected by the weather. When the sun comes out, most of us feel rejuvenated, but

those who continue to battle demons are reminded that they are different—not hopeful, and once again alone.

William Falk, editor in chief of *The Week*, noted, "Much of the
year, Finland has but a few hours of light, and temperatures well
below 0 degrees F. Yet the Finns are the happiest people in the world
according to the U.N.'s annual World Happiness Report."[68] The next
three countries on the happiness scale, the report says, are Norway,
Denmark, and Iceland. Like Finland, they are cold and dark during
much of the year. Meanwhile, the United States ranked eighteenth.

When it comes to day of the week and time of the year, suicides
and homicides are "perfectly out of sync with each other," notes
David Lester. "Homicide spikes not on Mondays but on the weekends." Homicides also spike on national holidays, unlike suicide,
and during summer and winter months rather than during
spring.[69] Another difference is that homicide rates are highest in cities, while suicide rates are highest in rural areas. People in cities
live close together, tend to be strangers, and often have substantially
different economic means—all potentially leading to conflict. Conversely, people in rural area are more spread out, know their neigh-
bors, and are more likely to have similar lifestyles. Rural areas have
less access to services such as hospitals, clinics, mental health agencies, and the like, however. They also have a greater percentage of
men, especially white men, and greater preponderance of guns.

As for the weather, a study of 866,000 suicides in the United
States and 74,000 in Mexico found a correlation between warming
trends and suicide. The study, which was conducted by Stanford
University and the University of California at Berkeley, found that
hotter temperatures result in more suicides—as many as 40,000
more in the two countries—representing a 0.7 percent increase in
the suicide rate in the United States and a 2.1 percent increase
in Mexico.

To further prove the point that weather has a direct influence on
people's mental state, and consequently contributes to thoughts of

suicide, the same researchers evaluated more than 600 million Twitter posts. They determined that every 1.8-degree Fahrenheit increase in temperature (or 1 degree Celsius) resulted in a 1 percent greater likelihood that the tweet was depressive in nature, containing words such as *lonely* or *suicide*. This mirrored almost exactly the correlation they found between increased suicides and hot weather. Researchers noted that when they analyzed the tweets by gender and economic status, they found no difference between men and women or rich and poor.[70]

Inasmuch as suicides have been increasing in recent years, as have the effects of global warming, the study raises the strong possibility that the two—climate change and suicide—are related, and not in a small way. In fact, the report concludes that when it comes to suicide, the effect of increased temperatures is "comparable to the estimated impact of economic recessions, suicide prevention programs, or gun restriction laws."[71]

More studies are needed to confirm this, but it's one more thing for everyone to worry about as icecaps melt, sea levels rise, and "natural" disasters such as droughts, floods, and fires become increasingly common.

Suicide and Covid-19

In 2022 an assistant professor at the University of California, San Francisco, School of Nursing wrote an opinion piece in the *San Francisco Chronicle* titled "No, I'm Not 'Fine,' and There Are Millions Like Me." She started by saying, "I spent my early twenties eying bridges, subways, high-rise windows, and busy traffic corridors, assessing which one would provide the most assured escape from my mental pain." Treatment for severe depression "helped save my life," but two decades later "depression has crept back as I've shouldered pandemic fatigue, grief from my father's death, and accumulated work and caregiver burnout."[72]

Other health care professionals and caregivers have experienced the same sense of despair and mental exhaustion arising from Covid-19 and its variants, as have millions of people in general. According to a psychologist writing in *Psychology Today*, the first suicide connected to the virus occurred in Italy in March 2020, when a male patient who was waiting for the results of tests regarding whether he was infected jumped out of a hospital window. "Since then," the author states, "numerous other suicides have been reported, primarily among front-line health workers, people awaiting test results, and those who have been affected by coronavirus-related bankruptcy."[73]

One high-profile suicide was a state finance minister in Germany, who despaired over the monetary effect of the virus. Another was a Manhattan emergency room physician who was on the front lines treating Covid-19 patients.[74] In the middle of 2020, the trauma director at John Muir Health, a large medical provider in my area, was interviewed on ABC-TV. "We've seen a year's worth of suicide attempts in the last four weeks," he said.[75]

A variety of factors created a "perfect storm," said three psychologists writing in *JAMA Psychiatry*.[76] These included social isolation and staggering unemployment rates, both directly tied to suicide. On top of this, gun sales have surged in the United States. Since access to firearms is a major risk factor for suicide, it's reasonable to think that the already high number of firearm-related suicides will increase even more.

Tom Bartlett, a reporter with the *Chronicle of Higher Education*, doesn't necessarily agree. Writing in 2021 in the *Atlantic*, he said, "The evidence supporting a broad, pandemic-driven suicide crisis among teens—or adults, for that matter—was always a narrative in search of data."[77] He pointed to the fact that for every Clark County, Nevada, where the *New York Times* reported that eighteen students had died by suicide from mid-March 2020 to the end of December— twice the number for all of 2019[78]—there were parts of the country that had reported a decrease. In Marin County, California, for instance, suicide deaths dropped by 33 percent, from 46 in 2019 to 31 in 2020.[79] These kinds of fluctuations happen from year to year, Barrett said, and to draw conclusions at that point was premature. Moreover, while being isolated from friends or in an abusive home can increase the risk of suicide, being out of school can protect kids from bullying and reduce their ability to access drugs and alcohol. Also, just because someone is stressed doesn't mean that he or she is suicidal.

The Crisis Text Line partners with the 988 Suicide and Crisis Lifeline and other entities to prevent suicides. In the spring of 2021 the organization issued a report, "Everybody Hurts 2020." It said that beginning in March with the pandemic, and continuing for the rest of the year, anxiety and stress had replaced depression and suicide as the top issues among 850,000 people in 1.4 million text conversations. In fact, conversations in which texters expressed thoughts of suicide dropped by 20 percent in 2020, compared with 2019, according to the report, which added, "This trend was also noticeable in the relative drop in conversations flagged as 'at imminent risk of suicide,' where a texter indicated they were thinking about ending their life, and they also had a plan, the means, and wanted to make an attempt within 48 hours."[80]

In 2019 there was a slight dip in the number of suicides nationwide, and it continued into 2020. The number of people who died by suicide in America in 2020 was just under 46,000, which was lower than the numbers in 2017, 2018, or 2019 but higher than in any other previous year. Suicide rates in the United States rose by 4 percent in 2021, however, to nearly 48,000. They rose again in 2022, to a record 49,449. The overall increase was 3 percent, but it was much higher for people 65 and older (8 percent) and people aged 45 to 64 (7 percent).[81]

The suicide rate among men—23 per 100,000—remains four times as high as the rate for women—6 per 100,000. According to the CDC, for every person who died by suicide in 2021, there were eight suicide-related hospitalizations and twenty-seven suicide attempts. Once again, firearms were used in more than half of all completed suicides.[82]

The CDC also reported that in the first seven months of the pandemic, US hospitals experienced a 24 percent increase in mental health–related emergency visits for children aged 5 to 11 and a 31 percent increase for adolescents aged 12 to 17.[83] Knowing this, it's not surprising that the biggest increase in suicide deaths from 2020 to 2021 occurred among girls aged 10 to 14 and the second-biggest increase was among teenage boys and young men aged 15 to 24.[84]

It's too early to know the full effect of Covid-19 on the suicide rate in the United States and elsewhere, mainly because it takes time to study things like this. It's important to note, however, that ending suicides represents a greater challenge than does neutralizing Covid-19. The answer isn't as straightforward as a vaccine, and there aren't the same financial incentives. It's daunting, but like the virus, it's surmountable if we as a society put our hearts, minds, and resources into it.

CHAPTER 4

Special Situations

ACCORDING TO THE CENTERS FOR DISEASE CONTROL AND PRE-
VENTION, most people kill themselves at home. For them, suicide
is a private act. Also, if they have the means at home, it's the most
convenient place. Other people don't want family members or
friends to find their body. That is one reason why they kill themselves in remote locations, such as parks, or in a hotel room.

On rare occasions, suicidal people want to be seen. Ken Baldwin,
whom I interviewed for my book *The Final Leap*, said that he had
felt as though he had gone unnoticed his entire life and decided that
his death would be different. "Jumping from the bridge was going
to force people to see me," he said, "to see me hurting, to see that I
was a person, too."[1]

Miraculously, Baldwin was one of the few people to survive a
jump from the Golden Gate Bridge. Even more miraculous was
that he incurred only minor, temporary injuries. Today he is a
popular high school teacher, offering proof that it's possible for suicidal people to turn their lives around if given another chance.

Suicide in Parks

Parks are a popular place for people to kill themselves. On occasion, park rangers have intervened successfully to prevent a suicide; however, their ability to talk someone out of it usually is hampered by a lack of training, the large territory they oversee, and the small ratio of park rangers to park visitors. More often than not, they are summoned to an area after hikers chance upon a body.

While the vast majority of people frequent parks because they are attracted to nature, a tragic few seek neither solace nor grandeur. Instead, they go to parks with another purpose: to end their life. In an article on suicides in national parks, the Associated Press summarized a few of the deaths:

> A 46-year-old carpenter with cancer climbed into a canoe and vanished in Everglades National Park.
>
> A 49-year-old builder blamed the economy in a note he left for his ex-wife and attorney before killing himself at the edge of the woods at Georgia's Kennesaw Mountain National Battlefield Park.
>
> A 65-year-old university biology professor disappeared into Utah's Canyonlands National Park, telling relatives in a note he was returning 'body and soul to nature.'
>
> A 70-year-old woman left a suicide note in the trunk of her car at Arizona's Saguaro National Park before killing herself about a half-mile from a trailhead.
>
> Three people, in separate cases, jumped off a towering bridge at West Virginia's New River Gorge National Park.[2]

In December 2010, the CDC reported on suicides occurring in national parks from 2003 to 2009. There were 194 suicides plus 92 attempted suicides. Those might seem like small numbers given the magnitude of suicide in this country and the fact that the deaths were spread out over eighty-four parks; however, the impact of each suicide on park resources, staff time, and witnesses, not to mention victims' families, can't be overstated. Moreover, the CDC noted that the actual numbers no doubt are higher because some deaths are handled by local law enforcement, who don't always inform park rangers. In addition, there are parks so vast that bodies may not be found until they have decomposed, making it difficult to determine the manner of death.

According to the CDC report, 84 percent of people who kill or attempt to kill themselves in national parks are men. The most common means is a firearm, with jumps and driving off a cliff being favored by a smaller number of individuals. Summer is the most popular time, and the settings with the strongest allure—Grand Canyon National Park, Golden Gate National Recreation Area, and Colorado National Monument—have the highest rates.[3]

Each suicide or attempted suicide creates a financial burden for parks, as well as a psychological burden for rangers. Search-and-rescue operations can require dozens of people, cost up to $200,000 each, and take rangers away from other duties, such as enforcing park regulations, stopping speeders, providing first aid to hikers, building exhibits, leading interpretive programs, repairing trails, and managing campgrounds. If a search ends in body retrieval, the mental impact on everyone involved can be profound.

One prospective park ranger in North Carolina was asked during his job interview, "If a visitor killed himself in the park, and you were the first person to reach his body, are you ready to handle it?" The situation was common enough to prompt the question. He told a reporter later, "You're sitting there in your suit and tie, and you want to answer the way you know they want you to answer, but I had to stop for a second and say, 'Am I?'"

It turned out that shortly after being hired he was put to the test—twice. The first time, a man's dead body was found in a remote area of the park after his wife called police saying that her husband planned to kill himself and had left her a message with the name of the trail he would be on. After police and the coroner left the scene, the park ranger, using a flashlight, cleaned everything up so that visitors to the trail the next day would not know what had happened there.

A week later, the ranger was standing at the edge of one of the park's lakes teaching a group of children how to tie a hook onto a fishing line when a call came in that a park visitor had heard a gunshot and seen a body. Remaining calm, the ranger told the group that he needed to help someone who had gotten hurt, and he instructed the adult chaperones who were there to take over. Then he rushed to the scene, but like other would-be rescuers he was too late. The man was dead. Afterward, the ranger wondered whether he could have done anything to prevent either death, and he talked with close friends and family members in an effort to process the trauma he felt.[4]

There are no easy answers to the problem, but park rangers are being taught to ask people who look despondent, "Are you here to hurt yourself?" It's a jarring question, and for that reason it is often hard for a ranger to ask, yet critical. Rangers who have been trained in effective suicide prevention strategies know how to follow it up, how to establish rapport with the person, probe, get them to a safe place emotionally, at least temporarily, and connect them with resources. Rangers also are being taught to look for notes taped to steering wheels, which seems to be more common in parks than in other locations. In addition, some areas in parks are closed now at night, and physical barriers such as guardrails are being erected at certain locations.[5]

As for park visitors, they can help by following the advice of Andrew Gulliford, a professor of history and environmental studies at Fort Lewis College in Durango, Colorado: "When I visit my favorite national parks again this summer," he wrote in a Colorado magazine, "I've decided to pay attention to more than just the scenery. I'm going to look a little more closely at my fellow visitors. And if someone seems lost and lonely, maybe I'll offer to share a cup of tea or a beer and engage in some conversation. It's the least I can do, not just for them but to help to help our hardworking, compassionate Park Service rangers."[6]

Suicide in Prisons

The United States has the highest incarceration rate in the world. We imprison 716 out of every 100,000 people. Russia is second, with 450 in 100,000. Much farther down is every other country, with Norway (70), the Netherlands (69), Finland (55), Sweden (53), Japan (47), and Iceland (45) having among the lowest rates.[7] America also has the highest prison population, with more than 2.1 million people behind bars. China is second, with 1.7 million, followed by Brazil (659,000), Russia (624,000), and India (420,000).[8]

The primary purpose of prisons is to punish people for criminal acts. Secondary to this is removing dangerous individuals from the general population. There is little public interest in what goes on in prisons, and even less interest in prison suicides. Whether inmates kill themselves, are killed by other inmates, experience an accidental death, or die of natural causes while they are locked up is of little concern to nearly everyone on the outside. Only inmates' families care. For the rest of us, they are easy to ignore.

Yet as Graham Towl and David Crighton point out in their study *Suicide in Prisons: Prisoners' Lives Matter,* from a human rights perspective, and based on the values and beliefs of a just society, inmates deserve to be treated respectfully despite the wrongs they may have committed. In addition to meeting inmates' basic needs, this includes guarding them from themselves as well as from others. "There is a duty to preserve and protect the lives of those kept within state custody independently of what crimes they have committed," Towl and Crighton state.[9]

A large number of inmates have mental health issues. In California, my state, 30 percent of prisoners receive treatment for serious psychiatric conditions. Many others don't receive treatment, however, despite having a diagnosable mental disorder. Either they don't seek treatment or the prison doesn't have the capacity to provide it.[10]

For inmates with psychological disorders, their mental health deteriorates during incarceration. How could it not? Even the most resilient person would have a hard time living in a small cage, under constant watch by guards who are accustomed to using excessive force and surrounded by other inmates who would like nothing more than to harm them.

Male inmates are six times as likely to kill themselves as men in the general population. Women in prisons are twelve times as likely to die by suicide as women on the outside.

According to Towl and Crighton, both psychology professors in Britain who studied every prison suicide that occurred in the United Kingdom from 1978 and 2014—more than two thousand altogether—the risk of suicide is greatest during the early period of imprisonment, when a person's future looks the bleakest and adjusting to years behind bars is the most challenging. Even so, many prison staff receive no training in suicide prevention. That's not just prison guards, sometimes referred to as correctional officers, or COs, in the United States, or hospital staff in a prison. Towl and Crighton note that teachers and workshop leaders may spend more time with individual inmates than prison officials and thus be in a better position to sense an inmate's frame of mind than guards, who are considered by inmates to be adversaries. Little or no effort is made to train them, however.[11]

It's obvious, perhaps, but worth stating anyway that prisons don't house a random cross section of the general population. Instead, they house, by and large, the poorest and most disadvantaged members of society. Individuals who are undereducated, unemployed, homeless, mentally ill, and ethnic minorities are represented dispro-portionately. Many lack any kind of family support, either because they have abandoned their family or because their family has aban-doned them. Many, too, are victims of crimes as well as perpetrators of them.

The problem of suicides in prisons is compounded by the prac-tice of placing some inmates, generally those who are the most trou-blesome, in solitary confinement. According to Harvard professor Stuart Grassian, inmates held in isolation are the ones who are most likely to attempt suicide. Roughly one-third are "actively psychotic and/or acutely suicidal."[12] Their cells are smaller than 100 square feet—just big enough for a twin bed, a toilet, and a sink—and it's not unusual for inmates to be confined in them for twenty-three hours a day. They are let out just once for an hour to take a shower or walk the yard, often shackled and always accompanied by a guard. This can go on for weeks, months, or in the case of death row inmates, years. On a typical day, an estimated 80,000 to 100,000 adults in the United States are in solitary confinement.[13]

In 2011 Lindsay Hayes, a national expert on suicide prevention in prisons, was hired by California to analyze prison conditions in the state. He concluded that California's suicide-watch practices en-couraged inmate deaths by holding inmates for long periods of time in dim, airless cells with unsanitized mattresses. Also, guards—not mental health workers—determined many conditions of sui-cide watches, such as whether inmates were allowed to shower, and guards sometimes falsified watch log entries showing how fre-quently inmates were checked. Hayes analyzed twenty-five cases and determined that in seven of them inmates killed themselves soon after they were taken off suicide watch. After Hayes submit-ted his report, the key findings were suppressed so that, according to the *Los Angeles Times*, Governor Jerry Brown could continue to claim that California's prison crisis was over and inmates were re-ceiving timely and responsive mental health care.[14]

Six years later, the only thing that had really changed was that more mentally ill people in California depended on state prisons rather than community-based services to take care of them. The *San Francisco Chronicle* noted in a 2017 editorial that the average state prisoner costs California in excess of $70,000 per year—not including the cost of mental health care. By contrast, the cost of treating a mentally ill person in a community-care setting was $22,000. "Unfortunately, California has a severe shortage of community-based mental health treatment facilities," the editorial said. "The state's total number of short-term, acute, psychiatric-care beds, for example, has decreased 30 percent since 1995." The editorial concluded, "Until California takes its investments in mental health seriously, the state's mentally ill will have to settle for the housing and treatment they can get. The fact that this housing and treatment is increasingly in the state prison system shames all of us."[15]

Compounding the problem of long wait times for mental care, high vacancy rates for prison psychiatrists, and a lack of suicide-prevention training for staff, prisons often fail to monitor inmates with suicidal tendencies, fail to refer sick inmates for a higher level of mental care, and respond to inmates who express a desire to hurt themselves by placing them in isolation cells. In these cells, inmate clothing often is removed and replaced by a safety smock, which resembles a full-body oven mitt and serves as clothing, a blanket, and mattress all in one.

Said one inmate, "Their idea is to wrap you in a mattress suit and put you in a cell by yourself until you don't have these feelings anymore."[16] He and others maintain that nothing is done to combat the frequent bouts of extreme isolation and feelings of hopelessness that inmates have. Moreover, the fear of being put in an isolation cell is strong enough to discourage many inmates from seeking help.

It's not just California. In 2018 forty inmates in Texas prisons killed themselves, the highest number in twenty years.[17] It's also not just prisons. Jails house thousands of people who are awaiting trial or serving short sentences, and they do not always house them well. There are roughly 3,100 jails in the United States. In 2019 the Associated Press and the University of Maryland's Capital News Service jointly investigated 165 lawsuits brought in recent years against local jails regarding inmate suicides and suicide attempts. The jails were charged with refusing to give inmates medication to manage their mental illness, ignoring inmates' cries for help, failing to properly monitor inmates, and imposing conditions that were excessively harsh.

Suicide has been the leading cause of death in US jails for years, but in 2014 it hit a high of 50 deaths for every 100,000 inmates, two and a half times the rate in state prisons and three and a half times the rate among the general population.[18] More recent statistics aren't publicly available, but with the suicide rate continuing to climb nationally and the number of people being locked up showing no signs of decreasing, it's safe to assume that the situation hasn't improved.

A 2010 study by the National Center on Institutions and Alternatives, commissioned by the US Department of Justice, analyzed 696 jail suicides over a two-year period. The NCIA found that 24 percent occurred within the first twenty-four hours of incarceration, and another 27 percent in the first fourteen days. Hanging was far and away the most popular method, used by 93 percent of inmates, which is no surprise given that bedding was the only means the majority had access to. A large number—38 percent—were being held in isolation, yet only 8 percent were on suicide watch at the time of their death.[19]

Suicide in the Military

There are a variety of ways to break down and analyze military suicides. One is by separating suicides of active-duty service members from those of veterans. Another way is to differentiate between vet-

erans of the war in the Middle East and veterans of previous wars—
Vietnam, Korea, World War II. A third way is to look at the difference between suicides of active-duty service members who deployed
and experienced combat and suicides of those who never deployed.
A fourth way is to compare active-duty service members in one of
the four military branches—Army, Navy, Air Force, and Marines—
with reservists and National Guard members. Lastly, one can focus on each branch of the military on its own.

In broad terms, since the so-called war on terror began in 2001,
four times as many service members and veterans have killed themselves as have died in battle.[20] It's "something to think about before
you or your child sign that dotted enlistment line," says one veteran
of the wars in Afghanistan and Iraq. "A soldier, sailor, airman, or
Marine is four times more likely to die by their own hand than by
the enemy's."[21]

For a long time, military leaders said that the number of service
members who killed themselves mirrored the number of suicides in
the general population once demographic factors such as age and
gender were considered. The majority of service members are men
aged 20 to 24, and this is also one of the highest-risk age groups
among civilians. It was a convenient argument to make because
prior to 2000 the military didn't track suicides by active-duty troops
or veterans, so it was difficult to disprove. Since 2000, however, data
have been available, and the results are clear.

For veterans generally, males have a suicide rate that is two times
the rate for males who aren't veterans. The rate for female veterans
is six times the rate for female civilians. Among veterans aged 18 to
29 the disparity is even greater. The suicide rate for males in this
group is nearly five times as high as the rate for male nonvets the
same age, while female veterans aged 18 to 29 have a suicide rate
that is eleven times the rate for their civilian counterparts.[22]

It's difficult for someone who has never served in the military,
much less experienced combat—myself included—to understand

what it's like to be deployed today. Troops face the constant threat of dying or being seriously injured. They witness violent deaths and the maimings of others. In addition to the grief they feel following the death of a friend in the service, they often feel responsible for it, believing that they didn't do enough to protect the person. There is also survivor guilt, guilt because they lived while their buddy didn't. Lastly, they feel that no place is safe. Even when they are behind concrete walls in a forward operating base (FOB), they are subject to mortar fire at any time. This is why they carry their weapons everywhere, including into latrines.

A study of troops in Iraq found that 94 percent had been shot at, 68 percent had seen dead or seriously injured Americans, 51 percent had handled human remains, 48 percent had killed an enemy soldier, and 20 percent had killed a civilian.[23] Given these experiences, it's hardly surprising that many troops are traumatized. This is especially true of National Guard members and reservists, who in recent years constituted half or more of the US fighting force in the Middle East. Most of them didn't enlist with the intention of participating in combat, but they deployed anyway.

Something that relatively few civilians think about is that the way war is waged has changed, increasing the psychological stress on troops. Today's battlefields are asymmetrical, meaning that there is no front and no rear. Every person in a war zone is at risk. There is no time to relax, because troops must be on guard every second. This need for constant vigilance and hyperalertness—referred to by troops as 360/365; that is, it's all around them every day—takes a toll and leads, among other things, to sleep deprivation and a reliance on medications to function, further putting active-duty service members at risk of suicide.

In addition, the distinction between enemy combatants and civilians has become blurred. Uniforms aren't worn by insurgents, and often woman and children are used as shields or as suicide bombers. American troops must decide in seconds whether to fire on someone who might be innocent—or might not. As I noted in my book *The Last and Greatest Battle*, and quoting the Reverend Rita Brock, who has consoled many mentally damaged service members, "There are no good choices. If you're looking at a kid on the side of the road with something in his hand, if it's a grenade and he throws it and kills someone in your unit, you've failed your comrade. But if it's a rock, you've just shot a kid with a rock."[24] The same was true in Vietnam, but that war was fought mainly in jungles. The conflict in the Middle East, however, which continues in some places, has been waged primarily in urban settings, exposing more civilians to harm.

Another factor is that the role of American troops today is much broader than in previous wars. US service members have been responsible for directing traffic, running prisons, maintaining utilities, and building schools, tasks for which they often have received little or no training.

Finally, there is the increased number of reservists and women in our fighting force. Both groups are alienated from other members of the armed forces, reservists by virtue of that fact that they live off-base and aren't full-time military, and woman by virtue of their gender, which makes them targets of sexual assault. According to an analysis of sixty-nine studies in the journal *Trauma, Violence & Abuse*, nearly one-fourth of women in the military report experiencing sexual assault, and more than half report harassment.[25] The fact that perpetrators often go unpunished and service women who report an assault often experience retaliation or receive a less than fully honorable discharge can result in female suicides. According to Defense Department data, women make up 16.5 percent of today's combat troops yet account for 31 percent of all suicide attempts by active-duty troops.[26]

The way a service member's military experiences play out affects not only that individual but his or her family. When service members come home from war, they often feel a need to make constant perimeter checks to ensure the safety of family members. They may hang security lights and get a guard dog for protection. In addition, they often try to limit outside activities of their spouse and children because they don't feel that they have as much control over what happens to them. At night they avoid lighted areas because they feel exposed. They also avoid dark areas, where the enemy can hide more easily. They avoid confined spaces like stairwells, where escape is harder, and crowded places like big-box stores, amusement parks, and farmers markets, because of the fear of a suicide bomber.

When it comes to driving, they are overly aggressive, tailgating and refusing to yield the right of way because their survival in the Middle East often depended on it. Many don't wear seatbelts because that hinders a quick escape. To dull their senses and numb their pain, they self-medicate with alcohol and/or rely on prescription painkillers. They also keep a loaded firearm nearby at all times because without it they feel defenseless.

These behaviors by themselves don't lead to suicide, but they add up. Inasmuch as suicide is for the most part an individual act, it's easy to blame the individual for not being tough enough, strong enough, or resilient enough to cope with his or her military experiences. After all, the vast majority of people who serve in the military do not kill themselves. Often, military leaders attribute a service member's suicide to the breakup of a relationship, a financial setback, a legal issue, or a drinking problem—all individual foibles. The focus is on providing more training in suicide prevention, as if individuals only need more training to end the problem, even though in many instances the problem didn't exist prior to the person's enlistment.

Training is the military's answer to everything. It's straightforward, relatively cheap, and what military service is predicated on. Suicide-prevention training isn't directed toward veterans, however, and less of it is provided to reservists and National Guard members. Moreover, when it comes to suicide, training is inadequate. To understand why, one need look no further than at suicides of active-duty service members who never deploy.

While it's understandable, perhaps, that service members who deploy and experience combat are at high risk of suicide because of the atrocities they witness and the psychological trauma they bring home with them, those who never deploy are also at risk. According to one study of service members who died by suicide between 2008 and 2011, 55 percent had never deployed and 84 percent had no documented combat experience.[27] Half the reservists and members of the National Guard who kill themselves have never deployed. How is this possible?

According to a 2011 report in *Suicide and Life-Threatening Behavior*, while deployment and combat exposure were factors, a more important factor was boot camp, otherwise known as basic training. It is in boot camp that troops learn to be tough and aggressive and not to show any sign of weakness. They learn to suppress emotions, deal with conflict through violence, become intolerant to pain, and be fearless in the face of death. These are the same qualities that make an individual more at risk for suicide.[28]

Developing ways to reverse this training once someone leaves the service and then implementing them are critical to ending the problem. As I note in the last chapter of this book, and explain in fuller detail in my book *The Last and Greatest Battle*, we can't just give troops pills and expect them to return to full health. Just as they have been trained for months to become fighting machines, an equal amount of training is necessary when their military service ends so that they can successfully transition back into civilian society.

Troops have easy access to lethal means. They learn how to handle all kinds of weapons, and after they leave the service they often keep firearms nearby for protection and security. Restricting access to lethal means is difficult in the military but not impossible.

In Israel the suicide rate for men aged 20 to 24—a high-risk group among civilians, and higher in Israel because of mandated military service—was reduced by 40 percent when soldiers no longer were allowed to take their weapons home on weekends. One small institutional change saved hundreds of lives.[29]

For veterans the solution is somewhat different. In 1789 President George Washington said, "The willingness with which our young people are likely to serve in any war, no matter how justified, shall be directly proportional to how they perceive the veterans of earlier wars were treated and appreciated by their nation."[30] Judging by this standard, we are failing. Many veterans who served their country with pride now feel abandoned. Their biggest challenge in transitioning to civilian life is receiving health care and compensation for injuries related to their military service.

Admittedly, the Department of Veterans Affairs has a huge mandate. Among other things, it's the largest health care provider in the country. Workloads are high. Even so, this doesn't excuse the fact that many veterans still wait months for their claims to be processed or to get a medical appointment. Some who can't wait any longer kill themselves.

Between 2016 and 2022, there were 2,279 suicides by active-duty service members, according to the Defense Suicide Prevention Office, or an average of 326 per year. Close to half (45 percent) were in the Army, with the highest number in 2020, the first year of the pandemic, although the number rose steadily from 2016 to that time. Marines made up 15 percent of the total, with the Navy and Air Force constituting 20 percent each. During the same period, there were 1,349 suicides by reservists and members of the National Guard, or an average of 193 per year.[31] The latter constituted 60 percent of the total, and the former 40 percent. Among both active-duty service members and reservists who died by suicide, firearms were the primary means.[32]

Assisted Suicide

As noted early on in this book, it's not a crime in the United States to kill yourself. It's a crime almost everywhere, however, to assist someone in killing themselves if you are not a physician and don't live in a state where physician-assisted suicide is legal.

Many Americans support the right to assisted suicide in cases of terminally ill patients who are in uncontrollable pain. When the time comes, each of us wants a "good death"—in our home, surrounded by loved ones, and in charge of our life up to the end. Often, however, people die in hospitals, surrounded by doctors and nurses who seemingly are in control. Court decisions have affirmed the right of patients to discontinue life-sustaining treatment. What is unresolved, though, at least in the majority of states, is whether people should have the right to enlist the help of doctors in hastening their death.

For many years, the right-to-die debate in America revolved around Dr. Jack Kevorkian, who maintained that adults with a terminal illness deserved to control the timing and manner of their death. Their years of experience gave them the necessary perspective, he said, to decide what kind of life they wanted and what kind they didn't want. This belief has been expanded in recent years by advocacy groups who cite the principles of empowerment and autonomy at life's end to justify aid-in-dying laws for people who aren't ill but are tired of living. They know what they want and what they don't want, so the thinking goes. Why should we interfere?

One otherwise healthy 65-year-old woman wrote in notes to a friend, "Can I be totally in love with this day of fall and not feel like I need to see every fall from now on? . . . Will my loved ones get that I may be done and that my passing is not personal." When she suffocated herself, she left a note for the coroner. "Call it a voluntary death," she wrote, attempting to avoid the stigma of suicide.[33]

The coroner didn't have a choice, though. In the United States there are only five accepted manners of death—homicide, suicide, accidental, natural causes, and undetermined—so he had to check "suicide."

Opponents of assisted suicide—and I am one—voice two main arguments. The first is that it's a violation of physicians' Hippocratic oath. According to the American Medical Association's Code of Medical Ethics, "Physician-assisted suicide is fundamentally incompatible with the physician's role as healer, would be difficult or impossible to control, and would pose serious societal risks."[34] Moreover, sanctioning physician-assisted suicide leads to a "slippery slope," says a 2020 editorial in *JAMA Internal Medicine*.[35] Do we draw the line with people who are terminally ill but mentally competent, or with people who, like the woman above, are competent but not terminally ill? What about someone who can't give their consent because of dementia or because they are in a coma? Where does it end? Dr. Guy Micco, of the Program for Medical Humanities at UC Berkeley, asks, "Do we become so inured to killing that we have involuntary euthanasia as in Nazi concentration camps?"[36]

The second argument is that physician-assisted suicide is an affront to people with severe disabilities, whose lives might seem to others not worth living. The message, say disability advocates, is that society may not support you and help you live, but it provides legal ways to get rid of you.

Opponents of assisted suicide, like Dr. Ezekiel Emanuel, chair of the Department of Medical Ethics and Health Policy at the University of Pennsylvania and former chief health policy adviser to the Obama Administration, point out that most people who seek euthanasia, according to studies, are motivated by psychological factors—primarily depression—not unbearable physical suffering. "The euthanasia debate has been carried on in almost total ignorance of the facts," Emanuel says.[37]

Assisted suicide became legal in Belgium and the Netherlands in 2002 for patients in "constant and unbearable physical or psychological pain" when attested by two or more doctors. Initially this meant cancer patients, but since then it has come to include people without a terminal illness. In 2014 Belgium included minors who had received their parents' permission to end their lives,[38] while in the Netherlands the age limit is 12, "providing there is strong medical evidence that psychiatric conditions have made their lives 'unbearable.'"

That policy came into question in 2019 when a 17-year-old girl told her ten thousand Instagram followers that she wanted to die after being sexually assaulted at age 11, raped at age 14, and suffering from anorexia and PTSD ever since.[39] It turned out that initial reports of her death erred, however, when they said that she was euthanized. In fact, she died after refusing all food and drink, and her parents respected her desire not to be force fed. Still, was it right that she was allowed to die, or did the country's health care system fail her? Is it always too soon to give up on a child, or are there exceptions? Do deaths like this motivate other young people whose lives seem unbearable to opt out early, or is every young person's suicide unacceptable?

To me, the answer isn't to assist people in dying. Rather, it's to improve end-of-life care so that people are better able to cope with depression, isolation, feelings of hopelessness, and a fear of burdening others. This way they have more reason to live.

In the United States at the time of this writing, physician-assisted suicide is legal in California, Colorado, Hawaii, Maine, Montana, New Jersey, Oregon, Vermont, Washington State, and Washington, DC.[40] It has been on the ballot in other states and no doubt will continue to be proposed. Worldwide, in addition to Belgium and the Netherlands, assisted suicide is legal in Canada, Columbia, Switzerland, and parts of Australia, and laws against it are being relaxed in Germany and Portugal.

Suicide by Cop

Suicide by cop is a form of assisted suicide. A person who wants to die brandishes a weapon at police with the goal—or at least the intent—that officers will shoot him in self-defense. (The use of the male pronoun is deliberate in this instance because suicide by cop is rare among females.) In some cases the suicidal individual may lack the capacity to kill himself. In other instances he may consider it more manly to die in a hail of bullets than to point the gun at himself and pull the trigger.

No one keeps statistics on suicide by cop, but there have been a few isolated studies. In one, researchers analyzed 437 instances between 1987 and 1997 in which police officers in greater Los Angeles shot and killed someone. Every death officially was ruled a homicide, although 46 fit the description of what researchers defined as "law enforcement-forced assisted suicide." All 46 individuals flashed a weapon at officers, but only half the weapons turned out to be loaded. Eight weren't even real guns; they were toys or replicas, although officers didn't know that at the time they fired their weapons. Forty-five of the 46 people were male. Two-thirds had talked of suicide to a family member or friend. More than one-third had a history of domestic violence. Nearly one-third had received psychiatric treatment at some point.[41]

In 2015 the San Diego District Attorney's Office issued a report on 358 officer-related shootings between 1993 and 2012. Nineteen percent were considered to be suicide by cop, but no details were provided other than the emotional impact on police officers, which can be traumatic. It's not like shooting a bad guy who has just robbed a bank, hurt someone, or fired at them first. Cops are trained to de-escalate situations in which a mentally ill or suicidal person is acting out, but that isn't always possible if an individual wants to be shot and forces the issue. There isn't time for cops to say, "Wait, can we talk about this?" or "Is that a real gun?"

According to one criminology and justice professor, suicide by cop "is completely outside the rubric of what policing is about."[42] That said, it's important to note that suicide by cop is different than police brutality cases, in which an unarmed person—almost always male and Black—is killed by cops in the course of attempting to flee a scene or resisting arrest or is just is in the wrong place at the wrong time. In those instances the victim doesn't want to die, whereas dying is the whole point for suicidal people who taunt cops into shooting them.

The psychiatrist Barry Perrou, a former crisis negotiation team commander and noted expert on suicide by cop, says that police officers need to be able to recognize persons exhibiting some common indicators. These include, most obviously, men who have just killed someone, particularly a close relative such as a mother, wife, or child, and who believe that they have nothing to live for or that they will be caught and imprisoned for the rest of their life. It also includes men who barricade themselves and refuse to negotiate with police or whose negotiations don't include any terms for their escape or freedom. In addition, men who have a record of assaults, who have experienced one or more traumatic events, such as the death of a loved one, a divorce, or financial ruin, and who say that they will only surrender to the person in charge are prime suicide-by-cop candidates. Then there are those who reference "going out in a big way," which is an overt indication of their intent.

Perrou also notes three behaviors that indicate a person's frame of mind and preparation to die. One is hypervigilance, in which the subject increasingly scans his surroundings and becomes more anxious, especially as additional first responders—police and paramedics—arrive. The second is a change in the subject's rate of breathing, either faster or slower, which may be evident visually, audibly, or both. The third is a practice of counting, up or down, sometimes in cadence with a rocking motion. Anytime one or more of these behaviors are observed, there is a heightened risk. The appropriate response, Perrou says, is for the police to interrupt with forceful words, telling the person to stop what he is doing and talk to them.[43]

Murder-Suicide

A murder-suicide is an act in which a person kills one or more people before taking their own life. In highly publicized cases, such as mass shootings at schools, businesses, and public places, or vehicular homicides on crowded city streets in which multiple people are deliberately run over, the horror looms large in the public consciousness. Most people don't think of these killings as murder-suicides, however. They think of them as murders, and the fact that the perpetrator kills himself at the end is relevant only insomuch as it spares victims' families from the emotions of a drawn-out trial, and taxpayers from the cost of years of incarceration.

Fewer than 2 percent of all suicides in this country, about eight hundred per year, are preceded by murder.[44] Most occur away from the spotlight, with relatively few people knowing about them. The overwhelming majority of murder victims in such cases —75 percent—are women, whereas 75 percent of the victims of homicides are men.[45] These murder-suicides often follow years of abuse and jealousy by the man, with alcohol usually playing less of a role than in other types of suicide.[46]

"One central theme seen in all types of murder-suicide," say the authors of a report published in the *Harvard Medical School Guide* in 1999, "is the perpetrator's overvalued attachment to a relationship that, when threatened by dissolution, leads him to destroy the relationship."[47] That relationship could be a marriage or romance, or it could be a job. Murder-suicides in which a fired employee returns to the workplace and shoots his boss and coworkers before killing himself have become, if not frequent, more commonplace today.

In *The Perversion of Virtue: Understanding Murder-Suicide*, Thomas Joiner breaks down the phenomenon of murder-suicide into four basic types. Each type is virtuous in the mind of perpetrators, Joiner says, because they believe they are doing the right thing, regardless what society thinks. Take the husband who shoots his chronically ill wife to take her out of her misery before he shoots himself. To others it's murder, but to him it's a mercy killing.

Then there is the wife who murders her abusive husband before killing herself. In her mind the act is just because she is righting the many wrongs that he committed against her. A variation of this is the spouse who kills her child before killing herself. Her justification is that she is sparing the child from a lifetime of pain and hardship at the hands of society in general or, perhaps, the child's father in particular.

In World War II, Japanese kamikaze pilots flew their planes into Allied warships to try and sink them. (The word *kamikaze* means "divine wind" and refers to a typhoon in the thirteenth century that destroyed an enemy fleet.) They didn't have a death wish; rather, they considered it their duty, which strikes some people as crazy. It's not that different, though, from a soldier who single-handedly rushes the enemy in an ill-fated attempt to kill as many as he can, or someone who jumps on a live grenade to save others in his unit.

Today there is the seeming madness of terrorists and suicide bombers who, much like kamikaze pilots, are willing to sacrifice their lives to a cause. Rather than being driven by a sense of duty, however, they are motivated by religious doctrine that life on earth is merely a prelude to eternal afterlife and they will be revered forever for what they have done.

Some murder-suicides, Joiner says, involve more than one type of virtue. He notes that the two teenage boys who killed thirteen people at Columbine High School in Littleton, Colorado. before killing themselves had reportedly been bullied by other students, particularly athletes, so justice in the form of revenge seemed to be their motive. Yet none of the people they killed were athletes. Based on journals and videotapes that they left behind, their primary goal was glory—to kill more people than the Oklahoma City bomber, who had been responsible for 168 deaths in the worst nonmilitary massacre in the United States prior to 9/11.[48] (That might have happened at Columbine if the bombs they planted around the school hadn't malfunctioned.)

Not all murder-suicides conform to these four types, Joiner admits. A few mass murderers, for instance, seek neither justice nor glory, aren't duty-bound, and have no sense of compassion or mercy. They also don't intend to die. After realizing that they can't escape, however, and not wanting to face the consequences of their heinous acts, they kill themselves. This makes them different from the norm, if it's possible to consider any norm for murder-suicides, because in other cases the perpetrator knows well in advance that he will die in the course of carrying out his plan. Moreover, he accepts it, after which he may give it only fleeting thought. His focus, after all, isn't on self-preservation but on the deaths of others.

CHAPTER 5

Talking to a Suicidal Person

FOR MANY PEOPLE, SUICIDE IS MORALLY REPREHENSIBLE. It's against their religion, against their culture, or contrary to their personal values. Talking about suicide, like other unpleasant subjects—incest, disease, discrimination—is avoided. Some people believe that individuals who want to die should be allowed to do so, that if they feel that their life no longer has meaning, that they are tired and worn out, or that they are a burden to others, they should be able to let go with society's blessing, or at least without any interference.

Overriding everything is the fact that suicide is so alien to most people—after all, the goal is to live a longer life, not a shorter one—that they believe it's impossible to dissuade someone who is intent on dying. This is a product of our Western culture, which emphasizes rational thought. We assume that all human behavior, including suicide, is rational even though sometimes it's not. Some people are more likely to develop a mental illness than others, but all of us, regardless of age, gender, race, culture, religion, sexual orientation, or socioeconomic status, have the potential to kill ourselves if our life spins out of control. This is what makes suicide so terrifying, that the sudden death of a loved one, an unexpected layoff, a financial crisis, or myriad other calamities can change one's outlook in a second. As a society, we are afraid to acknowledge this, however, so instead we assume that suicidal people are different. We distance ourselves from them in order to protect ourselves from a reality we don't want to confront, much less accept.

Given this, it's understandable why suicide isn't talked about and why we don't show those who are contemplating suicide or who have attempted it the compassion people usually show toward others. The prevailing sentiment is: Why bother? Why invest time, energy, and resources in preventing people from doing something that seems unpreventable? In the United States today, with industry and technology all around us, with freeway overpasses, tall buildings, and bridges to jump from, and train crossings to jump to, with an abundance of firearms that can be purchased virtually anywhere, with over-the-counter drugs sold in bulk at thousands of places for quick and easy consumption, it's easier to take one's life now than ever before. Why not just let people do it? It's legal, after all. Allow the rest of us time to turn our heads so we don't have to look, and one can make a permanent exit.

The answer, quite simply, according to those who know, who have lost a loved one to suicide, is because if it were your son or daughter, sibling, parent, spouse, partner, or friend who was holding a loaded gun, stepping into a noose, or climbing over the railing of a tall bridge, you would want them to be saved. If you were there, and there was no physical reason for them to want to die, you would try desperately to talk them out of it. If you knew that your loved one planned to end his or her life, you would do anything to stop the attempt. Wouldn't you?

Risk Factors and Warning Signs

While suicidal behavior is complex, thoughts of suicide often result from problems that seem unfixable. Gambling losses, legal issues, relationship problems, academic failures, mental disorders, unemployment, substance abuse, grief, and feelings of being a burden to loved ones can contribute to insurmountable feelings of despair—but not for everyone. Some people are able to manage these challenges, while others can't, and that is more difficult to explain. Just as two people may experience the same horrific event and yet only one of them develops PTSD, two people can experience similar setbacks and yet only one of them resorts to suicide. Is it because the other one has stronger coping skills and is more resilient? Few, if any, of us could withstand the tragedies faced by Job in the Bible, whose livestock, servants, and ten children die and who is made to suffer from horrible skin sores (all to prove his faith in God), but most of us have had to bear our own heavy burdens. If they don't push us over the edge, is it because we are able to find a bright side somewhere, to hold on to something positive even in the midst of an overwhelming loss? And if we can find something, why can't others?

It's true that some people give no indication that they are thinking of killing themselves. The vast majority do, though, in their words and in their actions. In assessing for risk, counselors focus on the following factors, which increase the likelihood of a suicide attempt:

- One or more previous attempts
- A mental disorder
- Substance abuse (alcohol and/or drugs)
- A family history of suicide
- A loss of any kind (of a loved one, relationship, job, pet, financial security, house, mobility, independence)
- Physical isolation and disruption of social support networks
- Ready access to a firearm
- A debilitating illness

In addition, counselors probe for warning signs:

- Talking about suicide or making statements revealing a desire to die
- Drastic changes in behavior (apathy, moodiness)
- Withdrawing from family and friends
- Losing interest in hobbies and in personal appearance
- Ongoing depression (chronic crying, sleeplessness, loss of appetite, feelings of hopelessness)
- A sudden change from extreme depression to being "at peace"
- Worsening academic or job performance
- Lack of interest in activities and surroundings (dropping out of sports and clubs)
- Settling affairs (giving away prized possessions)
- Increased irritability or aggressiveness
- Remarks suggesting profound unhappiness, despair, or feelings of worthlessness
- Death and suicidal themes in written work
- Self-destructive behavior (taking unnecessary risks or increased drug or alcohol use)

There is a myth that people who talk about killing themselves won't really do it. This is wrong. Before attempting suicide, many individuals make direct statements about their intention to end their life or less direct comments to the effect that they might as well be dead or that their family and friends will be better off without them. Any reference to suicide should be taken seriously. People who have already tried to kill themselves are especially at risk, even if their previous attempts seemed halfhearted or designed more to gain attention than to inflict self-harm. Unless they are helped, they may try again, and the next time could be fatal.

In asking questions and assessing intent, it's important to avoid making false promises and comments that might add to a person's dark mood. For example, saying that a lover probably will return or that someone's depression will go away may serve to lift someone's spirits temporarily, but ultimately it might result in an even harder fall if the promise doesn't materialize. In the same way, telling someone that they are better off than most people and that they should appreciate how lucky they are only increases feelings of guilt and makes the suicidal person feel worse.

Many suicidal people have given up hope, believing that they can't be helped. Most likely, though, things will improve for them at some point if they are able to hang on. Bad times, like good times, don't last forever.

Asking the Question

It's hard for most medical professionals to ask whether a patient has ever considered or attempted suicide and whether they are considering it currently. Many doctors and nurses haven't been trained to do this, don't know what to look for, and don't know how to create an effective suicide-prevention plan. Therefore, they shy away from asking about suicide. The same is true for many therapists. Although they may have more experience than doctors in talking with clients about mental health issues, they might lack training in suicide prevention.

Given how hard it is for professionals to ask about suicide, it's even harder for family members, friends, and colleagues. Just saying the word *suicide* can be difficult. "I understand that asking about suicidal thinking is scary," wrote a developmental psychologist whose teenage daughter had killed herself three weeks before her high school graduation, but "it is even scarier for the teenager who is thinking about it."[1]

The famed suicidologist Edwin Shneidman maintained that in dealing with suicidal people, the only two questions any helper needs answers to are "Where do you hurt?" and "How may I help you?" Subsequent experts have decided that that isn't enough, though. Helpers need to put aside personal fears regarding the answer and ask directly about suicide: "Are you thinking of killing yourself?"

It might be somewhat less scary to ask, "Are you thinking of hurting yourself?" or to say, "I hope you're not thinking of killing yourself," but these aren't nearly as effective. The former introduces euphemisms into the conversation, which lead people to talk around the problem, while the latter alludes to the helper's discomfort in talking about suicide, which discourages openness and honesty. Asking directly about suicide relieves the anxiety of a suicidal person who has been afraid to talk about how they are feeling. The person now has permission to unburden themselves.

When the person does start to talk, crisis counselors can assess the immediate risk of suicide—whether an attempt is imminent or the person is still ideating. The counselors probe, ask more questions, determine what supports the individual has to get them through the crisis, and discuss potential options that lead to a plan. A common technique is called "active listening," whereby the listener affirms what the caller is feeling and avoids making judgments. No one's pain is ever alleviated by criticism. Even if our words are intended to be constructive, or we think we know a person well enough to be frank, we can never know everything they are thinking or feeling. Fortunately, we don't need to. We only need to care, to let them know that we care, and to help them find reasons to go on.

To do this, helpers must focus on the moment. They need to ask themselves what they can do right then, in the next minute, or in the next hour. They need to be present, committed, and compassionate, the way they would want someone to be if the roles were reversed and they were the person dealing with suicidal thoughts.

In assessing the risk, a number of other questions are woven into the conversation:

"Have you thought about how you might do it?"

"Do you have access to a gun or pills or a jump site?"

"Have you thought about when you might do it?"

"Is there someone you can talk to?"

"Does your therapist know how you're feeling?"

"What do you think he or she would say if you told them?"

"How long have you been feeling this way?"

One of the phrases helpers sometimes use to encourage suicidal people to develop a different mind-set is, "Suicide is a permanent solution to a temporary problem." This is something that I said more than once early in my career, before I learned that it's flawed. It may apply to some youths who are depressed and contemplating suicide, but it's less applicable to older people, for whom there is an irreversible decline in mobility, vision, hearing, physical health, mental health, and the number of friends. In addition, a professional career might be winding down or have ended, resulting in fewer connections, reduced finances, and diminished self-esteem. These are permanent challenges, not temporary ones, and the depression that sometimes results from them isn't easily lifted.

Dr. David Jobes is a clinical psychologist who has treated hundreds of suicidal patients. One question that he suggests all mental health professionals ask of anyone who is suicidal is, "When you think of suicide, does it scare you or comfort you?"[2] The fact is that the thought of suicide can be comforting to people who feel trapped in their own self-described hell. It's a coping strategy to employ if someone's pain becomes too great. The suicidal person's perception of the world has become so constricted by his or her suffering that nothing else matters. People who are experiencing mental, physical, or emotional anguish aren't likely to relinquish the thought of suicide. They know that if the pain becomes unbearable, they have a way out. What helpers try to do is expand the person's perspective. They talk about who will find their body, loved ones who will be left behind, and the potential lessening of the person's pain over time. Individuals continue to have the freedom to make their own decisions, including the decision to end their life, but options are presented.

In his book *Danger to Self: On the Front Line with an ER Psychiatrist*, Dr. Paul R. Linde writes, "For the average person, it may seem hard to believe that many people keep suicide on their list of possible coping strategies should their pain become too great." Paradoxically, though, "keeping it on the list is the one thing that prevents them from actually doing it."[3] He cites the case of a bipolar writer who said that she had "no grand wish for death" and didn't view suicide "as a desire to end life or a dramatic way to go down in flames. Rather, it is a tool in my possession—the only one, really—that offers a permanent end to my pain. . . . That, I tell myself, is my earned choice."[4]

To a suicidal patient Linde says, "I understand you're not likely to take suicide off your list, but I'd like you to push it from second or third place back down to seventh or eighth or, better yet, fifteenth."[5] The option is still there, but it's not the only one. One psychologist says the same thing a little differently: "As a tactic, I ask the suicidal person to actually convince me that suicide is the only option left."[6]

In *Definition of Suicide*, Edwin Shneidman describes counseling a college student who was single, deeply religious, and pregnant. The woman was overcome with shame and had decided to kill herself. "I did several things," Shneidman said. For starters, he took out a piece of paper and began to "widen her blinders." The conversation started with Shneidman saying that the woman could have an abortion locally, to which she replied, "I couldn't do that." He said that she could go elsewhere and have an abortion, and she said, "I couldn't do that." He suggested that she could bring the baby to term and keep it, prompting the same response, "I couldn't do that." Alternatively, he said, she could have the baby and adopt it out. Again the woman said, "I couldn't do that." Shneidman said that they could get in touch with the young man involved, or involve the help of the woman's parents, and the woman said, "I couldn't do that." He ended the listing of possible options by saying that she could always kill herself, but there was no obvious need to do it that day. The woman, for the first time, was silent.

"Now," Shneidman said, "let's look at this list and rank them in order of your preference, keeping in mind that none of them is perfect." The very making of the list had a calming effect. "Within a few minutes," Shneidman says, "her lethality had begun to de-escalate. She actually ranked the list, commenting negatively on each item. What was of critical importance was that suicide no longer was first or second. We were then simply 'haggling' about life—a perfectly viable solution."[7]

The Advent of Technology

At one time, the prevailing opinion among many mental health professionals was that suicide hotlines wouldn't be effective. "Several issues arise when using the telephone as the primary venue for assessing a patient's psychological functioning," said four clinicians writing jointly in the journal *Suicide and Life-Threatening Behavior*. "Assessing and diagnosing patients without seeing them in person deprives the clinician of important clinical information such as body language, eye contact, appearance, posture, and grooming. In addition, it is difficult to manage a crisis when large distances separate clinician and caller. . . . Most importantly, it is difficult to develop a therapeutic relationship during a one-time telephone conversation."[8]

That didn't stop a small group of people from starting a suicide hotline in Los Angeles in 1962, nor did it stop a onetime priest and longtime San Francisco radio correspondent for the BBC from starting a suicide hotline in San Francisco the same year. The Los Angeles hotline was launched in part because of all the attention around Marilyn Monroe's death and was answered by professionals. The San Francisco hotline, by contrast, started as a one-person affair. Acting on a hunch, Bernard Mayes placed ads on Muni buses in San Francisco that read, "Thinking of ending it all? Call Bruce," followed by his phone number. Then, working under the pseudonym Bruce, Mayes answered calls on a couch in his basement. In the beginning he had no idea whether the phone would ring, but it did— once the first night, ten times the first week, and two hundred times the first month. Today, San Francisco Suicide Prevention answers two hundred or more calls a day from a high-rise downtown.[9] In time, more suicide hotlines sprang up around the country, each answered by local people, some who were experienced clinicians and others who weren't. It has only been in the past twenty years, however, that there has been a single, national phone number for suicide prevention.

In 2005 the National Suicide Prevention Lifeline, run by a non-profit organization based in New York City with funding from the federal Substance Abuse and Mental Health Services Administration, began operating what is today the country's primary suicide hotline. Anyone who is either suicidal or worried about someone who is suicidal can contact the Lifeline twenty-four hours a day, 365 days a year, for free, confidential counseling and emotional support. Calls are routed to roughly two hundred crisis centers accredited by the American Association of Suicidology, generally to the center that is closest geographically to the caller. Active-duty service members, veterans, and their families who call the Lifeline can press "1" to be connected to a center that has special expertise in military issues.

In July 2022 a new, national three-digit phone number—988—was instituted for suicide prevention, supplanting a ten-digit number (1-800-273-TALK), although that number remains active too. The organization rebranded itself the 988 Suicide and Crisis Lifeline, and the federal government granted it $282 million. The majority, $177 million, is being used to bolster the existing network of operations and telephone infrastructure, which includes text and chat response, as well as a subnetwork for Spanish-language speakers. The remaining $105 million is being used to build up staffing at local call centers.[10] In addition, many states provide matching funds.

It's not unusual for communities with robust crisis centers to keep their local number and use the Lifeline number as backup, although this may change with the advent of 988 if for no other reason than to eliminate confusion. Suicide-prevention hotlines, according to one definition, "provide phone-based services for individuals who are at risk of suicide or concerned about someone at risk of suicide."[11] That sounds fairly specific, but as the Rand Corporation reported in a 2016 assessment of California suicide-prevention hotlines, it overlaps, or at least appears to overlap, with other phone-based services. For instance, county governments in California operate Access lines that provide information and referral services to mental health consumers. There are also 211 lines, which provide information and referral for local health and social service needs and sometimes receive suicide calls. In addition, there are "warmlines," which assist callers in noncrisis situations. How calls are handled among the three varies widely, as do staffing requirements, counselor training, telecommunications equipment, hours of operation, protocols, call volume, and financial stability. Implementation of 988 may change that.

Three questions that the Lifeline recommends counselors ask callers are: "Are you thinking of suicide?," "Have you thought about suicide in the past two months?," and "Have you ever attempted to kill yourself?" Recommended follow-up questions include: "Will you talk to your therapist about this?," "If not, will you let me talk to him or her?," "Have you considered changing therapists?," and "Will you promise me to call here again if you're feeling down?"

At some point in the conversation, a caller might ask if the counselor will break confidentiality, trace the call, and summon police, an ambulance, or a mobile crisis unit to intervene if a suicide attempt seems imminent. The Lifeline's position is that counselors should be truthful, and this is the practice among participating crisis centers. One recommended response would be, "Yes, but only as a last resort, and we're not close to being there yet."

Having to hospitalize someone without their consent and holding them in a psych ward for up to seventy-two hours isn't a positive outcome from a counselor's point of view. It means that counseling failed, and once someone is released, they are unlikely to call the hotline again if they should have suicidal thoughts. They don't trust it, and being stopped from attempting suicide isn't, in the words of David Lester, "a beneficent act if it means that the person has to continue living a life that he hates."[12] The best solution is for the counselor to work with the caller to develop a specific safety plan. Not only does the plan get callers through the current crisis but it can keep them alive long afterward.

Counseling someone over the phone might not be as desirable as meeting with them in person, but it's effective nonetheless. Moreover, in one way it's more effective because clients have greater control. They don't have to worry about offending anyone if they walk out of a session; they can simply hang up. The physical separation also makes some clients more willing to share their troubles. In addition, clients can talk in the comfort and convenience of their home or office, so counseling is more accessible.

In recent years, crisis centers have begun offering text and chat services as well, sometimes in collaboration with Crisis Text Line, an independent agency that was started in 2013 by two women in New York City. Initially, the same concern was raised: that because the counselor could not hear the caller's voice, counseling would be ineffective. This too is proving to be untrue. While from a counselor's point of view a written conversation is less desirable than a phone conversation, which in turn is less desirable than talking to someone in person, it's better than nothing. Moreover, since texting is the preferred means of communication for many people, particularly youths—the average teenager sends nearly two thousand texts per month and 98 percent are opened compared with only 25 percent of emails[13]—it makes sense for counseling to be available to them this way. At the time of this writing, according to the Crisis Text Line website, nearly 9 million messages have been received since the service was founded, with 20 percent suicide-related. (Other common precipitators are relationship issues [38 percent] and depression or sadness [37 percent].)[14] Protocol requires that texts be responded to within five minutes by a counselor who is trained not to move into problem-solving mode too quickly.

On the plus side, texting affords more privacy than a phone call, as Alice Gregory noted in her 2015 *New Yorker* article on the Crisis Text Line, "R U There?" "Tears go undetected by the person you've reached out to," Gregory writes, "and you don't have to hear yourself say aloud your most shameful secrets."[15] The result is that people are more likely to disclose sensitive information about themselves in a text than over the phone. Teens might be strongly resistant to talk but garrulous when texting.

One challenge for providers is learning the abbreviations and emojis that make up a fair amount of texting. A counselor doesn't need to adopt the same written tone as the texter—and probably shouldn't—but the counselor needs to be able to understand what someone is saying. It's also critically important, for obvious reasons, that the counselor type carefully.

Hotline Counselors

One thing that always surprises people is that volunteers who answer hotlines at nationally accredited crisis centers are better trained and more experienced in dealing with suicidal people than most mental health professionals.

"Hotline counselors are not hesitant to discuss the difficult issue of suicide," the noted suicide expert David Lester says, "and they are able to talk directly about the caller's desire to die." By comparison, "many psychotherapists are ill at ease with suicidal clients and fear that they will be at fault if their clients complete suicide. This anxiety is partly due to the fact that most therapists see relatively few clients who are suicidal and, therefore, have little experience in this area. Telephone counselors, after working with large numbers of suicidal clients, soon become well acquainted with the issues involved. They acquire a vast fund of experience in working with suicidal and distressed clients, and so become quite skilled in helping them."[16]

The training that hotline volunteers receive is one reason why they are better prepared to help suicidal people than most licensed professionals, who, if they receive any training at all, are likely to focus more on pharmacology than on therapy. *JAMA*, the *Journal of the American Medical Association*, reported that 91 percent of physicians believe that their knowledge of suicide assessment and treatment is insufficient.[17]

Another reason is that volunteer counselors want to be there. No one is paying them, and they aren't in a rush to help a backlog of people. They stay on a call as long as they need to, as long as it's helping someone. Calls from actively suicidal people often last an hour or more, and a counselor has to develop rapport with callers and build their trust before developing a safety plan with them. There aren't any shortcuts for this; it's a process.

By contrast, the measures in place at some hospitals to prevent suicides emphasize restraint and medication but may offer little in the way of therapy. Around-the-clock observation, surveillance cameras, and seclusion rooms, where sharp objects and anything that can be used to form a noose are removed, don't help people deal with their problems and sometimes don't even prevent suicides. According to one source, about 5 percent of all suicides occur in mental hospitals, with half taking place during the first week of admission.[18]

One thing that counselors need to know is the caller's age. With seniors, a counselor might talk about ways to increase the person's social connectedness through volunteering, joining a service club, taking continuing-education classes, or adopting a dog, all of which give people a reason to get out of the house regularly. The conversation is focused on the present, on how to make things better now.

Conversations with youths also start out focused on the present but inevitably shift to the future. Referring to the caller's age can be an effective way to put their pain in perspective. Think of it this way, two Israeli psychologists say: "In killing the 19-year-old Ron, you will also be killing the 20-year-old Ron and the 30-year-old Ron and the 40-year-old Ron. You will be killing also the Ron that will perhaps be a father and grandfather. How can you choose for these other Rons, for a Ron that will be stronger and more mature? How can you choose for the Ron that you could become, but to whom you refuse to give a chance?"[19]

Often, if a phone counselor asks someone, "Why do you want to kill yourself?," the person answers, "It's a long story," as if they don't want to go into it and the counselor probably doesn't want to hear it. This may be the last—literally the last—call that the person ever makes, though. When a person dials a suicide hotline, it's a call for help. Part of the person wants to die, but another part wants to live, or else they wouldn't have called. Counselors focus on the part that wants to live.

"That's okay," the counselor says. "I'm not going anywhere. Tell me your story." This opens the door to a conversation, during which the counselor can learn how things got to be so hopeless for the caller and assess the caller's degree of pain. Callers feel pushed into a corner, emotionally and psychologically, and it's the counselor job to help them get out.

Survivors of Suicide

One of the confusing phrases in the suicide prevention world is *suicide survivor*. Someone unfamiliar with the phrase might assume that it means a person who has survived a suicide attempt. In fact it refers to a person who has survived the suicide of a loved one. This is no small feat, in part because suicide survivors are at higher risk of suicide themselves but also because the stigma of losing a loved one to suicide is so great.

"I used to drive down the street thinking I had a sign on my car that said MY SON KILLED HIMSELF," says Iris Bolton, who coauthored with her father a book about her 20-year-old son's suicide, *My Son . . . My Son . . . : A Guide to Healing After Death, Loss, or Suicide.* "Another car would pass me," Bolton says, "and I would think, 'Now they know.'"[20]

Many husbands and wives whose spouses kill themselves feel a similar loss of identity. They are no longer themselves but the widow or widower of a person who took his or her life. If they have lost children, they are no longer parents. Whenever they are out in public, they feel as if everyone is watching them, casting furtive glances and making whispered comments.

Anytime someone dies, it's traumatic for survivors, even when they have had time to prepare for it. Sudden deaths are more traumatic, and if it's a murder, the trauma is magnified. In many respects, however, suicides are the most traumatic of all, partly because they are usually sudden and often violent but mainly because of the guilt and stigma attached to them. Survivors think back on every interaction they had with the deceased, especially recent ones, questioning what they did or didn't do—all of the "what ifs." Did they miss warning signs? Did they take something the decedent said too lightly? Were they slow to act or did they not act at all, even in the face of what, in retrospect, was ominous?

Accompanying guilt is another strong emotion—anger. There is anger at the deceased for rejecting and deserting them. There is also anger at other family members and mental health professionals because they didn't prevent the suicide, whether they actually could have or not. There might even be anger at a higher being for letting it happen.

These feelings, along with sadness, loneliness, and depression, can be defeating. Dealing with them constructively is at the heart of grief counseling. Survivors may never fully recover from the suicide of a loved one—what passes as normal is different from what used to be considered normal—but it's possible to reach a point where the way the person died doesn't overshadow the way they lived and are remembered. Usually this starts when the survivor accepts that the reason why the person killed themselves may never be known, at least to the survivor's satisfaction. Continuing to expect an answer only delays the healing process.

There is another kind of suicide support group, for people who make an attempt and live. In the parlance of the profession, they are referred to as *suicide attempt survivors*. Support groups for them are rarer, in part because leading this kind of group is daunting. Not only is everyone in it at high risk but many suicidal people have emotional needs that can be overwhelming for the facilitator. This doesn't mean that group members are weak, though. "People assume that if you've struggled with suicide, you're fragile," said the program director of a statewide crisis and peer support group in Colorado. "But if you've struggled with this and you're still here, then you must be really strong."[21]

Typically, members of suicide attempters' support groups focus on their thoughts about suicide rather than on suicide itself. They talk about the dark moments in their lives that led them to attempt, coping strategies that have worked for them, and resources that they are familiar with—both good resources, such as a helpful service or therapist, and bad ones, like time spent in a psych ward. Individuals share things with the group that they don't feel able to talk about with other people in their lives, and in the process they often begin to feel more empowered and less stigmatized. "Talking doesn't change the event," said one suicide attempter, "but it can change how I feel about it and can make me feel less alone."[22] "People who swim together don't tend to drown," according to the executive director of a suicide-prevention center in New York.[23]

The same can be said when people who have experienced the epitome of despair don't hold it in anymore but talk openly and freely about it, especially with people who have been there too. Building connections is the basis of most support systems, and it requires a level of trust that enables people to feel comfortable letting down their guard and being vulnerable.

"I once read that we all have a prosecutor in our head who points out the things we've done wrong," said one suicide attempt survivor, "but we don't all have a strong defense attorney. Mine had gone missing entirely. I'd wake up at 3 A.M. and lie there thinking of all the ways I was defective. . . . That's what depression does—it lies."[24]

The writer William Styron, in *Darkness Invisible: A Memoir of Madness*, decried the word *depression* as being insufficient to convey the depths of someone's torment. A better description, he said, is "the veritable howling tempest in the brain."[25]

Styron had the presence of mind to check himself into a hospital when he was entertaining thoughts of suicide, and he survived to write about his suffering, but many others are reluctant to seek help. Instead, they hide their thoughts, ashamed about having them and unwilling to let others know, especially loved ones, who they believe won't be able to deal with them effectively and will sit in judgment besides.

"My children knew how to 'stop, drop, and roll' if their clothes were on fire," said one woman whose 15-year-old son had taken his life. "They knew to 'buckle up,' to 'just say no,' and to avoid 'stranger danger.' We had talked about drinking and driving, safe sex, and about substance abuse, but it had never occurred to me to talk about what depression feels like. Beginning that conversation is prevention."[26]

For loved ones, there are five things they should do and five things they shouldn't, according to David Lester. They should listen actively, ask direct questions, try to determine the degree of suicidal intent, seek professional help for the person, and follow through if the person doesn't. What they shouldn't do is appear judgmental, beat around the bush, deny a suicidal person's feelings, leave the person alone if the risk of suicide is high, or try to be a hero and deal with the situation on their own.[27]

It might seem like a lot to remember, especially in a highly stressful moment, but Lester's dos and don'ts have value beyond suicide prevention. They are a reminder that everyone is more than a diagnosis or a problem. "See the person, not the illness," is a common mantra in the mental health world. It's not easy to do sometimes, especially in cases where a person's depression, schizophrenia, manic episodes, or dementia tends to dominate their life, but helpers are most effective when they follow it. Unfortunately, there are no magic words. There is just the willingness of others to be present, listen, express concerns, and show that they care.

Suicide-Prevention Training

Several years ago the American Foundation for Suicide Prevention sponsored a magazine ad. The ad featured a photo of a good-looking young man in a white T-shirt sitting on a park bench. Printed on his T-shirt in large, black letters were the words "I'm suicidal." Underneath the photo was the headline "If only it was that easy to identify."

Medical doctors are trained to identify symptoms, diagnose problems, and provide appropriate treatment, all within the context of a physical ailment or condition. With the exception of psychiatrists, however, many physicians know relatively little about suicide. Their ability to probe into a person's psyche, deduce a problem, and treat it effectively is limited. People generally are more willing to talk about physical problems than they are mental ones. Unless doctors probe into a person's mental state—something most docs aren't comfortable doing—key risk factors are ignored and key warning signs are missed.

As noted in an earlier chapter, 75 percent of people who die by suicide visited their primary-care physician in the previous year. Nearly half visited their primary-care physician in the previous month. There are opportunities for doctors to ask about a patient's mental health, but they have to be trained to do it.[28] Many mental health professionals need training too. This is because in most states, psychologists, therapists, and clinical social workers aren't required to take any classes in suicide prevention to attain or retain a license. Training in suicide prevention is an option, and some choose it, but unlike training in child abuse, elder abuse, and domestic violence, it's not mandatory.

Whenever legislation has been proposed that would mandate suicide-prevention training for mental health professionals, licensing organizations have tended to oppose it. Even when the training would be relatively minimal, such as six hours of coursework for a first-time license or to renew a license and a refresher course every four years, organizations have fought it. The reason isn't that they think training in suicide prevention is a bad idea; it's that they feel they are subject to enough mandates already. They prefer to keep suicide-prevention training as an elective rather than a requirement, despite the dramatic and growing number of suicides in this country.

For individuals who do opt for training, there are a number of programs to choose from. One of the most popular is Applied Suicide Intervention Skills Training, or ASIST. Created by a Canadian agency called LivingWorks, ASIST is taught in communities throughout the United States, as well as in other countries. It's the training program that is endorsed by the federal Substance Abuse and Mental Health Services Administration, the US Army, and 988 Suicide and Crisis Lifeline. The training is intense, two full days with two trainers, and isn't limited to professionals; anyone who is interested can sign up for it. Almost without exception, people who complete the training say that they feel confident that they can help a person who is suicidal.

One of the elements in ASIST is a diagram that is referred to as the "River of Suicide." The river cuts through diverse landscapes—a city, a suburb, farmland—and ends in a waterfall. It serves as a metaphor for providing first aid to individuals who are suicidal. People enter the river at different times and from different locations. If they don't get help, they can end up at the waterfall, which signifies a suicide attempt. The point of the diagram is that suicide prevention doesn't start at the waterfall; rather, it happens all along the stream.

Another LivingWorks training is called safeTALK. It's a four-hour, face-to-face workshop on suicide prevention that combines presentations, audiovisuals, and practices. Participants learn basic skills such as how to recognize warning signs, engage someone, and connect them to appropriate resources for further support. Like ASIST, it's open to all.

QPR is slightly different yet also popular. The letters stand for "Question, Persuade, and Refer," three key steps in preventing a suicide. It's a takeoff on CPR (cardiopulmonary resuscitation), which is designed to stabilize people who aren't breathing, are breathing intermittently, or are experiencing cardiac arrest until professional help arrives. The goal of QPR, like CPR, is to be part of a "chain of survival" according to the QPR website, to increase a person's chance of surviving a mental or emotional crisis. Individuals determine the degree of a person's suicidal intent by asking questions, persuading them to get help, and referring them to resources for longer-term care. As with ASIST, QPR training is open to anyone, with the emphasis on gatekeepers. A gatekeeper is someone who is strategically positioned to recognize and refer someone at risk of suicide, such as a teacher, a minister, or a coach. It also can be a police officer, a gun shop owner, a firefighter, a paramedic, a military squad leader, or a caseworker. Through QPR, gatekeepers learn to recognize the warning signs of suicide and how to intervene effectively to save a life. The training is three to six hours, although some training is offered online.

Washington State, where the QPR Institute is based (Spokane Mental Health was an early partner and continues to provide funding and support) has been at the forefront of suicide-prevention training in the United States. In 2014 state legislation began requiring psychologists, other licensed mental health professionals, marriage and family therapists, drug abuse counselors, and social workers to take six hours of suicide-prevention training. In 2016 other health care professions—physicians, physician assistants, nurses, physical therapists, and chiropractors—were added. In 2017 the requirement kicked in for pharmacists, and by 2020 it included dentists and dental hygienists.[29] By instituting the requirement and also expanding it to include professions that don't often come up in conversations about mandated training, Washington is a model for other states.

Another source of training is the Suicide Prevention Resource Center. It's based in the University of Oklahoma Health Resources Center but conducts training around the country. In-person training for assessing and managing suicide risk is six and a half hours and aimed at behavioral health care staff who work in clinical settings. Other courses are online and open to anyone, although they are designed for mental health staff. One two-hour course focuses on preventing suicides in hospital emergency departments. A second course focuses on reducing a suicidal person's access to lethal means. A third helps people locate and understand data pertaining to suicide prevention.

The Media's Role

Following the deaths of the celebrity chef Anthony Bourdain and the fashion designer Kate Spade within days of each other in June 2018, suicide became a temporary topic of conversation. Numerous statistics were noted, including 44,965 (the number of people who died by suicide in 2016, the most recent year for which data were available at the time), 28 percent (the increase in the US suicide rate from 1999 to 2016), and 70 percent (the increase in the suicide rate from 2010 to 2016 among girls).[30] Alarms were raised about suicide being a growing yet still largely invisible public health problem. *The Week* called suicide "America's hidden epidemic,"[31] while an article in *Time* magazine on the deaths of Bourdain and Spade had the headline "Things Are Never What They Seem,"[32] and an editorial in the *San Francisco Chronicle* was titled "The Worlds We Fail to See."[33]

The *New Yorker* writer Andrew Solomon, whose own mother died by suicide, said that when people who are famous kill themselves, it captures our attention for two contradictory reasons. First, "it assures the rest of us that a life of accolades is not all that it's cracked up to be." At the same time, it forces us to ask, "How can our more ordinary lives hold up?"[34]

An early reviewer of this book voiced much the same concern. He said that we look to other people for problem-solving strategies when we feel that our own skills are lacking. Inasmuch as suicide represents a problem-solving strategy that others have employed to end their pain, it's an option. If the person who dies is a celebrity or otherwise considered to be successful, the thinking could be, "If they didn't want to live, with all that they had, why should I? If suicide was the answer for them, maybe it's the answer for me."

This is why the way the media covers suicide is critical. While individuals add to the problem by spreading rumors and false information, sometimes knowingly and sometimes not, news of a suicide often starts with reports in the the mainstream media, especially if the person who dies is well known, the circumstances are unusual, or there is a series of suicides by people who live in the same area and die the same way. The latter is referred to sometimes as the Werther Effect, after Johann von Goethe's 1774 novel *The Sorrows of Young Werther*. The title character, a young man who dresses in the style of the day, is angst-ridden because his love for a married woman is unrequited. In despair he kills himself, leading to a string of real-life suicides by young men who kill themselves in imitative fashion.

The history of suicide is replete with instances of copycat behavior. In 1792, a soldier hanged himself from a beam at Les Invalides in France. Within weeks, twelve other soldier hanged themselves from the same beam. When the governor closed access to that particular corridor, suicides ended. Similarly, in 1813 a woman hanged herself from a tree in the Swiss Village of Saint-Pierre-Monjau. Shortly thereafter, other women hanged themselves not only from the same tree but from the same branch.[35] In chapter 8 I note the suicide of a young Japanese woman who in 1933 jumped from an observation point into a volcano. Subsequently, nearly one thousand other people did the same thing.

In 1974 a sociology professor at UC San Diego led a team of students in analyzing front-page stories on suicide in three major newspapers and subsequent changes in suicide rates. In twenty-seven of thirty cases they found that the rate was higher than expected, with the most notable case being that of the actress Marilyn Monroe. After she killed herself, suicides in the United States increased by 10 percent the following month. Researchers determined this by comparing suicides in August 1962, the month that Monroe died, with suicides in August 1961 and August 1963.[36]

A 2002 report in the *Journal of Epidemiology and Community Health* analyzing forty-two separate studies on the impact of publicized stories about notable suicide deaths reached the same conclusion. It stated that there was a strong statistical correlation between media coverage of celebrity suicides and subsequent increases in the suicide rate generally.[37] A study by the Centers for Disease Control and Prevention found that suicides in the United States rose by 10 percent in the four months after the actor Robin Williams's suicide in August 2014.[38]

A related study was conducted by a professor in Vienna. As the radio show *Freakonomics* noted, in the 1980s there was a significant increase in suicides and suicide attempts on the Viennese subway. One person jumped in front of a train in 1983. The following year there were seven subway suicides in Vienna. Each was reported in graphic fashion in Austrian newspapers. In 1985 ten people jumped and died (three other jumpers lived). In 1987 eleven people died. After Austrian media were advised to tone down press coverage, refrain from including the word *suicide* in headlines, and not print photos of grieving family members, subway suicides and suicide attempts in Vienna dropped by nearly 80 percent.[39] The rash of train suicides in Vienna prompted a researcher at the Medical University of Vienna to study press coverage of suicide in five hundred newspapers. He concluded that the Werther Effect was real and that the way the media covers suicide had an impact on suicidal behavior.[40]

In Japan, an 18-year-old singing idol who was distraught over her relationship with an actor jumped from the top of a recording studio in Tokyo. In the next two and a half weeks thirty-three other young people killed themselves, many also jumping to their death. One of them had a photograph of the singer in his pocket, jumped from the same roof that she had jumped from, and landed on the shrine that her fans had created in her memory.[41]

It's not unusual after a student dies by suicide for other students in the same school or community to kill themselves, frequently in the same way. It's also not unusual for multiple troops in a battalion or platoon to take their lives following the suicide of one of their own. The phenomenon of suicide contagion, with one suicide leading to subsequent suicides, starts with how information about them spreads.

In this age of social media few things remain secret for long. Moreover, humans have a predilection for gossip that often results in misleading and factually incorrect information being disseminated rapidly, widely, and indiscriminately. People have a responsibility to verify the accuracy of anything they are about to tweet, post, or blog about. They also have a responsibility to consider the effect of their words on others.

In this regard, everyone would do well to follow the recommendations of the American Association of Suicidology to mainstream media regarding reporting on suicides:

- Avoid sensationalistic headlines or subject lines
- Avoid using graphic photos or videos
- Avoid explicit descriptions of how someone died
- Avoid simplistic explanations for the death

Instead of the headline "Kurt Cobain Kills Himself with Shotgun," for instance, news reports could say, "Kurt Cobain Dead at Age 27." Instead of photographing or filming the place where the death occurred, which only serves to draw people to the scene, the media can show the outside of a school or business where the person attended classes or worked but not the site of their death. Instead of images of grieving family members, which can be a source of revenge for individuals who haven't had good relations with parents or siblings, the media can use a yearbook, work, or family photo of the deceased. Instead of filming a well-attended memorial service, which can glorify the death in such a way as to lead others to imagine a similar outpouring of affection at their own death, the media can focus on close-ups of the printed program, a minister speaking, and floral arrangements while featuring a local crisis line number or the number 988. Although choosing pictures with less emotional impact is contrary to the way the media usually operates, it is critical when covering suicide.

Also important is the way the death is talked about. Instead of saying that someone's suicide is inexplicable, was impulsive, or happened without any previous indication of intent, media stories should include warning signs of suicide and information on what to do if someone you know exhibits these signs. Instead of reporting that someone's suicide was preceded by a single event, such as the recent loss of a job, the breakup of a marriage or a relationship, or bad grades, reports should say that suicidal behavior is complex and usually is the result of multiple causes, including psychiatric illnesses that may not have been recognized or treated.

Too often, reporters cover a suicide in the same way that they cover a crime. Suicide isn't a crime, however. It's a public health issue and should be covered as such, with background information on trends, rates, treatment options, and resources. Equally important, a person's suicide can be balanced with stories of hope and recovery in which suicidal thinking is overcome and skills to cope with adversity are increased. This way, individuals and the media don't unintentionally promote self-destructive behavior by contributing to suicide contagion but rather encourage people who are contemplating suicide to seek help.

At one time the Annenberg Public Policy Center analyzed the coverage of suicides in nine major newspapers over a period of twelve months, plus three years' worth of articles in the *New York Times*. Seven of the nine newspapers made a point of using the word *suicide* in at least half their headlines, sometimes in a sensational fashion. One headline in the *New York Times* was "Eighth-Grade Sweethearts in a Love Suicide." In many of the *Times*'s articles, the Annenberg Center found, the method of suicide was mentioned in the headline, yet only 8 percent of the articles cited depression as a possible factor in the person's death. Some of the journalists who were contacted by the center didn't know that certain types of news coverage can lead to imitative behavior, and none were aware that experts in the field had developed media guidelines for reporting on suicide.[42] That is changing—slowly—although it's still common for media reports to use the phrase *committed suicide*. Since the general public often takes its cue from the media, the use of this stigmatizing terminology needs to end.

PART II

RESTRICTING ACCESS TO LETHAL MEANS

CHAPTER 6

Guns and Suicide

THERE ARE THREE MAIN TYPES OF FIREARMS: handguns, rifles, and shotguns. The latter two typically are referred to as "long guns" because they have a long barrel, as opposed to handguns, which have a relatively short barrel and thus are more often used in suicides.

The estimated number of firearms in the United States varies depending on the source. According to production data from firearms manufacturers, 371 million guns are owned by private citizens and law enforcement personnel. Roughly 146 million of these are handguns.[1] The Centers for Disease Control and Prevention estimates that there are 650 million guns worldwide, and nearly half of them are owned by Americans.[2] According to a 2018 report by the Switzerland-based Small Arms Survey, civilians own 857 million of the world's guns, with Americans owning about 393 million of the total. That's 46 percent, even though the United States makes up only 4 percent of the global population.[3] A study by Harvard and Northeastern Universities puts the number of civilian-owned guns in the United States at slightly lower—265 million[4]—although that is still an average of more than one gun per adult. Of course, many individuals own multiple guns, while others, myself included, don't own any. According to national surveys, one-third of American households have a gun,[5] and 3 percent of households own half the total number of guns in the United States.[6]

There are many reasons for owning a gun. The primary one, according to gun owners, is for personal protection.[7] Lesser reasons include hunting and recreational or target shooting. Buying a gun specifically to kill yourself is far down the list; more often, the availability of a firearm provides ready access for someone who is contemplating suicide. Studies show that 83 percent of gun deaths in the home are the result of suicide, while only 2 percent are the result of an intruder being shot. Many of the suicides are by someone other than the gun owner.[8]

According to a 2022 report by researchers at Stanford and Northwestern Universities published in *JAMA Psychiatry*, women who live in households with a gun owner are 43 percent more likely to die by suicide than women living in gun-free households. The study followed 9.5 million women over twelve years. In the beginning, none of them lived in houses with a gun. That changed over time for 330,000 of them, however, as they came to live with a lawful gun owner. While the suicide rate for women who continued to live in a gun-free household didn't change, it increased dramatically for the others.[9] Another report, by Stanford researchers using the same data, found that women who personally owned handguns were seven times as likely to die by suicide as women who didn't own handguns. Despite the widespread belief that a gun in the home makes the inhabitants safer, researchers found the opposite to be true.[10]

An analysis reported in the *New England Journal of Medicine* of more than a dozen case-control studies in peer-reviewed literature reached the same conclusion: the risk of suicide in homes with a gun was two to ten times as great as the risk in homes without a gun.[11] *Bloomberg News* said the risk was three times as high.[12] Regardless which conclusion is the most accurate, the bottom line is that easy access to a firearm increases the risk of suicide.

The National Rifle Association continues to be one of the strongest lobbies in the United States, with more than five million members and a stranglehold on American politics when it comes to gun use. On its website the NRA lists five rules for gun safety: (1) always keep the gun pointed in a safe direction, whether loaded or unloaded; (2) always keep your finger off the trigger until ready to shoot; (3) always keep the gun unloaded until ready to shoot; (4) be aware of what is behind your target; and (5) never use alcohol or any drug, including prescription drugs, that might impair awareness or judgment when handling firearms. Beyond this, the NRA opposes virtually every law and action that attempts to implement other safety measures relative to owning a firearm or to limit the ability of private citizens to own firearms of any kind, including high-speed, military-style assault weapons. NRA officials cite the Second Amendment to the US Constitution as the foundation for their position, which states—somewhat clumsily, hence arguments about its intent—"A well regulated Militia, being necessary to the security of a free State, the right of the people to keep and bear Arms shall not be infringed."

James Madison, known as the father of the Constitution, was the primary author of the Bill of Rights. He also was one of three authors of the *Federalist Papers*, a collection of essays that explained the importance of the Constitution and why it had to be ratified. (Although the Constitution is treated with reverence today, from Supreme Court justices on down—sort of an American version of the Ten Commandments—it was strongly opposed by some at the time, making ratification far from certain.)[13] To appease people who feared a military uprising in the future, Madison and other framers of the Constitution said that it was important for private citizens to be armed. In *Federalist*, no. 46, Madison wrote that a federal standing army couldn't field more than 25,000 to 30,000 men and would be far outmatched by 500,000 armed citizens, thus negating the possibility of any kind of coup.

In the years since the Constitution was ratified, gun-rights proponents have argued that the Second Amendment recognizes an individual's right to keep and bear arms without restrictions, and US courts in general have agreed. Nevertheless, Madison might recoil at the way the amendment is interpreted today, says Dominic Erdozain, a theologian and researcher at Emory University. While it often is argued that the problem isn't firearms but who gets them, "the founders did not think this way," Erdozain says. "They did not divide the world into good guys and bad guys, darkness and light. 'If men were angels,' wrote Madison, 'no government would be necessary.' But they are not. . . . The minds that framed the Constitution had none of the gun culture's faith in the law-abiding citizen. . . . Mass shootings would not have surprised the founders. A government that tolerates them would."[14]

The Most Lethal Means

In 2005 *JAMA*, the *Journal of the American Medical Association*, published the most complete review to date of suicide-prevention strategies. Twenty-three physicians and scientists from the United States, Europe, and Asia authored the review after studying forty years of scientific research. They concluded that the two most effective ways to prevent suicide were to restrict access to lethal means and to train health care professionals to recognize suicide warning signs and intervene when the risk was present.[15]

Two facts about guns and suicide stand out. The first is that only 5 percent of all suicide attempts involve a gun.[16] Guns are the most lethal means of suicide, however. More than 85 percent of people who attempt suicide with a gun die as a result.[17] The reason why many suicidal people resort to a firearm is simple, according to researchers at Harvard's School of Public Health. Death is quick, and the effect is irreversible.[18]

Guns are used in more than half of all completed suicides. They are the most common means of suicide for males (56 percent) and tied with poisoning for suicides among females (31 percent). Farther down the list are suffocation (28 percent for both males and females), poisoning for males (9 percent), and other means (7.5 percent for males and 9.4 percent for females).[19]

By comparison, only 3 percent of drug overdoses are fatal, and the death rate for other methods of suicide is under 5 percent. If one swallows pills, inhales car exhaust, cuts oneself with a razor, or tries to hang oneself, there is time to reconsider, or time for another person to intervene. That isn't the situation with a firearm. "Once the trigger is pulled, there's no turning back," say Harvard researchers.[20]

In 2022 the Centers for Disease Control and Prevention reported that 48,117 lives were lost in America to gun violence, an all-time high. Suicides comprised the greatest number—26,992, or 56 percent—followed by homicides with 19,592, or 41 percent (the balance consisted of unintentional deaths and deaths resulting from law enforcement activities). Of particular note, while guns remain the leading cause of death for children and teens age 10 to 19, for the first time the gun suicide rate among Black children and teens surpassed the rate among white children. Overall, the gun suicide rate in 2022 represented a 1.6 percent increase from 2021, continuing a steady increase in the gun suicide rate from 5.55 in 2006 to 7.65 in 2022.[21]

Researchers studying the relationship between guns and suicide are quick to note that their message isn't against or in favor of guns; it's driven by facts. One might think that facts about suicide are readily available, but they're not. The CDC, for instance, in its National Violent Death Reporting System, collects information from police reports, coroner reports, and death certificates on suicides and homicides, but only in eighteen states. Results for the whole country are extrapolated. Moreover, it can take literally years before this information is complete. By comparison, the National Highway Traffic Safety Administration maintains a Fatality Analysis Reporting System, which receives data within thirty days for every fatal vehicle crash on US public roads, including weather conditions and whether drugs or alcohol were involved.

Is there a correlation between this diligence and the fact that in the past twenty years the fatality rate of car crashes has dropped by one-third? Matthew Miller, associate director of Harvard's Injury Control Research Center within the Public Health Department, thinks so. With better data, he says, "discussions are grounded in facts rather than distorted by ideology. . . . A public approach doesn't look so much to blame as to understand and present." He cites public relations campaigns about cigarette smoking, seatbelt use, and drunk driving as examples. "I'd like physicians to feel it's their responsibility to tell people about the risks. There's no reason that you should have a conversation about a bike helmet or a seat belt, but not firearms."[22]

There *is* a reason, though, as Miller and other people who study guns and gun violence know all too well. Researchers looking into other public health problems aren't subject to anywhere near the same level of scorn and ridicule by a powerful organization that lobbies Congress to defund it the way that people who study gun safety are. The closest parallels are tobacco companies and the pharmaceutical industry, both of which have considerable clout but not a single, vociferous, omnipresent voice like the NRA. Another difference is that with cigarettes and drugs, it's manufacturers who are leading the charge while with guns it's consumers. This is because smokers aren't as passionate about cigarettes as gun owners are about guns, while drug users are more interested in hiding their addiction than in calling attention to it. Following a 1993 report by the CDC stating that having a gun in the house tripled a person's risk of being shot by a family member or intimate acquaintance, the NRA lobbied Congress to include a restriction in the CDC's budget that none of its funding could be used to promote gun reform. Congress complied, and subsequently the CDC's budget for research on gun safety dropped by 96 percent.[23]

That kind of pressure means two things for people who want to study gun-related issues such as suicide. First, they have a difficult time getting funding to do it. Few private organizations grant money for this kind of work, and government funding for it is hard to come by given the NRA's opposition. Second, and perhaps even more daunting, they have to be prepared to have their credibility attacked loud and hard when their conclusions are published. It's one thing to study a public health problem that most people agree is significant but another thing to be verbally mauled by an influential organization with the ear of many elected officials. The result is that only a few institutions, most notably Harvard, have the financial wherewithal to pursue it and the academic standing to fend off criticism.

Harvard, to its credit, doesn't pull many punches. "In the U.S., where there are more guns, there are more suicides," say public health researchers.[24] It's that simple. To prove it, they compared firearm suicides in states that have the highest percentage of gun-owning households with states that have the lowest. Together the two groups comprised about 50 million people, with 47 percent of households having guns in the high group and 15 percent in the low group. After controlling for various factors, such as mental illness and drug and alcohol abuse, researchers found that rates of firearm suicides in states with a prevalence of gun owners were nearly four times as high as in states with the lowest rates of gun ownership (16,577 firearm suicides versus 4,257). It is notable that when the means of death was something other than a firearm, the rates for the two groups were virtually the same (9,172 suicides versus 9,259).[25]

To be clear, the reason for the difference between states with a high percentage of gun-owning households and states with a low percentage, say researchers, isn't that gun owners are more suicidal. "It's that they're more likely to die in the event that they become suicidal, because they are using a gun. . . . Changing the means by which people try to kill themselves doesn't necessarily ease the suicidal impulse or even the rate of attempts. But it does save lives by reducing the deadliness of those attempts."[26]

Mass Shootings

It might seem irrelevant in a book about suicide to talk about mass shootings; however, one thing that people often overlook is that many mass shootings end with a suicide. More often than not, the shooter turns the gun on himself, but sometimes police do the job in a scenario that is not very different from suicide by cop. It's a recurring theme of public mass shootings, says Sarah C. Peck, director of a gun violence initiative at Northeastern University School of Law, that the killers save their last bullet for themselves.[27]

Since the Columbine shootings in April 1999, mass shootings in the United States have become so common that Columbine no longer ranks in the top fifteen in terms of fatalities. Two of the worst mass shootings occurred in 2017. On October 1 a 64-year-old man broke out windows in his thirty-second-floor suite at the Mandalay Bay resort in Las Vegas and rained gunfire for at least ten minutes on twenty-two thousand people who were attending an outdoor music concert several hundred yards away. Fifty-eight people were killed, not counting the gunman, who subsequently killed himself, and five hundred others were injured in the worst shooting in Nevada history.

On November 5 a 26-year-old man killed twenty-five people and an unborn child during a Sunday service at the First Baptist Church in the small town of Sutherland Springs in southern Texas. Twenty other people were wounded. When it was over, the shooter was dead from a self-inflicted wound. It was the worst mass shooting in Texas history.

A year earlier, forty-nine people were killed, and more than fifty others were injured by a 29-year-old gunman inside a gay nightclub in Orlando. It was the worst mass shooting in Florida history, and then a year later seventeen people were killed at Marjory Stoneman Douglas High School in Parkland, Florida. More recently, in 2019 twenty-two people were killed in a Walmart store in El Paso, Texas, and fifteen hours later nine others died in a mass shooting in Dayton, Ohio.

Each tragedy has been different, but they share four similarities. First, one or more rapid-fire, high-capacity firearms were used that were relatively easy for the gunman to procure. Second, the people killed were, for the most part, strangers to the shooter. Third, the shooters were predominantly male and white. Last, in most instances the killer died of a self-inflicted gunshot wound—that is, suicide—before police could fire.

Each state where a major mass shooting occurred has reacted differently to it. In California, after the San Bernardino shootings the state began requiring background checks for the purchase of ammunition. In Connecticut, after the killings at Sandy Hook Elementary School the state banned high-capacity magazines. Conversely, in Virginia, after the 2007 shooting at Virginia Tech, which claimed thirty-two lives, not counting the shooter, the state loosened its polices, including no longer limiting purchases to one handgun per month. In Texas, after a mass shooting at Fort Hood the state began allowing licensed gun owners to carry guns openly in many public places. In South Carolina, following the June 2015 shooting deaths of nine African Americans at an Episcopal church in Charleston by a 21-year-old man who told police afterward that he wanted to start a race war, the list of states who honored other states' concealed-carry permits grew. As for Nevada, its policies are ironic, to say the least. Since 2012 it has been legal for a person to carry a real gun on the Las Vegas Strip but not a toy gun. Clark County commissioners approved an ordinance that bans flame throwers, blades more than three inches long, and toy guns in order to make the sidewalks safer, but there is no prohibition against actual firearms.[28]

It's worth noting, particularly in regard to mass shootings, that at the time the Second Amendment was drafted, it took fifteen to twenty seconds to load and shoot one bullet from a rifle. The most proficient infantrymen in the Civil War were able to fire only three shots per minute. That is a far cry from the automatic weapons of today, which can fire four hundred or more rounds per minute.

Also, when the Constitution and the Bill of Rights were written, only 14 percent of men owned guns, and half of those weapons weren't operable. A musket cost the equivalent of two months' pay, rusted if it wasn't properly maintained, misfired frequently, and was inefficient for self-defense or hunting because it wasn't accurate. Besides, most men were farmers and had no use for a gun.[29]

Michael A. Bellesiles, a Colonial historian at Emory College and author of *Arming America*, points out that the ownership of guns by private citizens, while common in Europe, didn't take off in this country until the 1840s. That was when Samuel Colt created a sighted pistol that could be aimed. Moreover, Bellesiles says, it wasn't until the end of the Civil War that gun ownership became an inherent part of American culture. Before then, guns weren't equated with freedom or independence; they were just weapons, and rather expensive and inefficient ones at that.[30]

We Are Number One

The United States is the only country in the world where guns are the primary means of suicide. In every age group except children aged 10 to 14, gun suicides outnumber all other forms of suicide.[31] (Among children aged 10 to 14, hanging is the most common means.)

Whether a person owns a gun and how he or she feels about guns tends to be a partisan issue. More than 40 percent of Republicans own guns, compared with only 20 percent of Democrats. In a 2017 poll by the Pew Research Center conducted, notably, several months before the mass shootings in Las Vegas and Sutherland Springs, fewer than one-third of Republicans said that gun violence was a big problem, compared with two-thirds of Democrats. In the same poll, when asked if there would be fewer mass shootings in this country if it were harder for people to legally obtain guns, 73 percent of Republicans said no, while 64 percent of Democrats said yes.[32]

The NRA maintains that the only thing that can stop a bad guy with a gun is a good guy with a gun. In 2014, however, the FBI studied 160 "active shooter" incidents and found that an armed citizen stopped the gunman only once.[33] According to Vox, only 3 percent of all mass shootings from 2000 to 2013 were stopped by an armed civilian. Moreover, "for every criminal killed in self-defense by a man, 34 people are killed in gun homicides, 78 people in suicides, and two in accidental gun deaths."[34]

Throughout much of the world, political leaders have concluded that there is a direct correlation between the number of firearms in circulation among the citizenry and the number of firearm deaths in the country. Several times after a single, horrific event has brought this issue to the forefront, commonsense gun laws have been implemented. In 1996 in Australia, for instance, the federal government banned all automatic and semiautomatic guns a month after thirty-five people were killed in a mass-shooting rampage. In addition, all firearms were required to be registered, and the government bought back seven hundred thousand guns from citizens.[35] The result was that the number of gun suicides in Australia dropped to half immediately—and has stayed there—while the number of suicides by other means hasn't increased. The number of gun homicides in the country also has decreased by half.[36]

In England and Wales, whose combined population is 56 million, relatively few people—only 6.5 percent—possess firearms. A major reason for this is that in the United Kingdom, as in Australia, there was a mass shooting in 1996. Thirteen children and a teacher were killed at Dunblane Primary School in Scotland by a 43-year-old man who subsequently killed himself. One of the students who survived the shooting was Andy Murray, who went on to become one of the world's top tennis players. Afterward, Great Britain banned military-style assault weapons and most handguns and confiscated 200,000 firearms and 1.4 million pounds of ammunition.[37] Since then the most common method of suicide in the United Kingdom has been hanging, followed by self-poisoning and overdosing. Gun suicides are rare. There are also relatively few gun homicides, fifty to sixty a year, or about one for every one million people. By comparison, the United States, which has six times as many people, has 160 times as many gun homicides.[38]

In Japan, gun ownership is virtually illegal, and homicide and suicide rates reflect this. Crime is so rare in Japan that often the police have nothing to do.[39] Japan does have a high rate of suicide, but not from guns. Asphyxiation, hanging, and jumping from a building or in front of a moving train are the most frequent means of death there.

In 2019 New Zealand banned automatic and semiautomatic weapons less than a week after a gunman killed fifty Muslims and injured at least fifty other Muslim worshipers at two mosques in Christchurch. The shooter wore a head-mounted video camera to live stream the massacre, and all five weapons he used, including two semiautomatic rifles with forty- and sixty-round magazines, had been purchased legally. New Zealand has a history of tolerance when it comes to private ownership of firearms, and at the time of the shooting there were 1.4 million guns in the country, which has a population under 5 million people. Nevertheless, Prime Minister

Jacinda Ardern moved quickly, with relatively no opposition, to implement the ban.

Then there is the example in Israel, noted in an earlier chapter, where in 2006 the Israeli Defense Force stopped letting soldiers take their weapons home with them on weekend leaves. The suicide rate dropped by 40 percent almost overnight, with no increase in firearm suicides on weekdays.

Contrast that with the United States. In recent years, especially during the Trump administration, the government denied any connection between the number of guns and the number of shootings. Indeed, the response was just the opposite: to advocate for arming more people with guns.

Deaths from firearms in the United States have been blamed on a variety of factors, from mentally ill people accessing guns to violent video games. Neither has credence, however. "People with mental-health disorders are more likely to be victims of violent crime than perpetrators, and more likely to hurt themselves than others," wrote two doctors in *Time* magazine in 2019. "Mental illness is certainly a problem in this country, but hate is not a mental illness."[40]

As for video games, of the perpetrators of thirty-three mass murders at US schools in the years 1980 to 2018, only four were known to be video gamers. A psychology professor at Villanova University who studies video games found that 70 percent of high school students play violent video games, but only a small fraction engage in actual violence. Researchers in Germany have spent years looking for a link between video games and violence but have found none.[41] Then there are the Japanese, who spend far more per capita on video games than Americans do but average fewer than ten gun deaths per year in the whole country.[42]

Supreme Court Justice Brett Kavanaugh has written that when it comes to guns, public safety shouldn't be a determining factor;

only "text, history, and tradition" matter, he says.[43] Given that belief, it's not surprising that he voted with other conservative justices to rule that gun owners have the right to take their guns across state lines, including to states that don't permit "open carry." "What other civilized country allows its citizens to show up, say, at a Starbucks carrying semi-automatic guns?" remarks one critic.[44]

It's all the more troubling because it no longer may be enough for states to pass laws that result in lower rates of firearm deaths. A neighboring state could undermine them. Nevada, for instance, has the loosest gun laws in the country, while California has the most restrictive. One study found a correlation between gun shows in Nevada and temporary increases in gun-related violence in nearby areas of California but no correlation between gun shows in California and spikes in gun-related violence in nearby areas of Nevada.[45]

As horrific as mass shootings are, the deaths don't always end there. Two teenagers who survived the 2018 shooting at Marjory Stoneman Douglas High School in Florida killed themselves in 2019. One had been diagnosed with PTSD, experienced survivor guilt, and said that she didn't feel safe in college classrooms.[46] The other was the father of a young girl who had been one of the victims in the mass shooting at Sandy Hook Elementary School. He also killed himself in 2019, after creating a foundation in his daughter's name to study links between mental health and violence. A week before his death, he met with parents of one Stoneman Douglas student.

Then there are the thousands of other people who escape mass shootings and have survived—so far—but continue to live with the trauma. "Twenty years after that day at Columbine High School, I'm still asking, 'Am I safe?'" says a graduate of Columbine who was a 14-year-old freshman when the 2012 shooting at the school occurred. Now a mother herself, she says that each time she drops her child off at nursery school with a hug, she has the same thought:

that this could be the last time she sees him. But that's not all. "The unexpected cold sweats, beating heart, and panic can come suddenly on a normal day—waiting in line at the grocery store, seriously taking notes on the exits in a movie theater. The thought: This is a shooting. How can I be safe? Twenty years later, I am still asking this question."[47]

According to a 2016 report published in *JAMA*, half the global gun deaths occur in six countries: the United States, Brazil, Colombia, Guatemala, Mexico, and Venezuela. Overall, of the 251,000 gun deaths worldwide in 2016, 64 percent were homicides and 27 percent were suicides.[48] This is different than in the United States, where more people take their life with a gun than are killed by someone else doing the shooting.

What the Gun Debate Is Really About

It's unlikely that the kinds of measures implemented in Australia, Great Britain, and New Zealand following mass shootings will be implemented in the United States, mainly because, as *Time* magazine reported in a 2017 cover story, "the debate over gun rights isn't really about guns at all. It's about what they represent: cherished freedoms, a reverence for independence. . . . Guns are a rejection of political correctness that creeps into everything. Even the most incremental move to constrain deadly weaponry seems to many Americans to cut against their rights."[49]

That may be true, but in poll after poll a large majority of Americans want stricter gun laws. This includes Republicans—79 percent of whom support background checks for gun shows and private sales, 78 percent of whom support laws to prevent mentally ill people from buying guns, and 55 percent of whom support a ban on assault-type weapons—as well as most Democrats.[50] Moreover, not all gun owners are opposed to all forms of gun reform. According to the Pew Research Center, 89 percent of gun owners believe that people who are mentally ill should be prevented from buying a gun, 82 percent believe that people on no-fly or government watch lists should be barred from buying a gun, 77 percent support background checks for those purchasing guns privately and at gun shows, 54 percent are in favor of creating a federal database to track all gun sales, and 48 percent support a ban on assault-style weapons.[51]

A poll by Quinnipiac University found even greater support for universal background checks: 97 percent of all voters, including 93 percent of Republican voters.[52] It's worth noting that the suicide rate in states with laws requiring universal background checks for firearm purchases is 53 percent lower than in states without these laws, and the per capita suicide rate is 31 percent lower.[53]

France has had more than its share of terrorist attacks with mass casualties, although most of these have involved trucks, cars, and bombs. One exception was in November 2015, when gunmen armed with automatic weapons burst into a concert hall and several restaurants in Paris, killing 130 people and wounding many others. None of the guns were purchased in France, however, because even though hunting is popular there, buying a gun in France is a process. Any firearm with a barrel shorter than 18.5 inches and a removable magazine that holds more than three rounds requires a sports shooting license, active membership in a shooting club, attending a firing range at least three times a year, and annual certification from a physician that the individual is physically and mentally fit to own a gun. Guns with longer barrels, such as those used primarily for hunting, also must be registered, and the owner not only must have a sports shooting license but also must take a full day of exams on gun safety and protected species. As a result of these measures, the number of privately owned guns in France dropped from 19 million in 2006, when the measures were implemented, to 10 million in 2016.[54]

Suicides in France also dropped. According to a study by the French National Suicide Observatory, there was a 26 percent decrease in the number of suicides in France between 2003 and 2014. That coincides fairly closely with the change in gun laws, although the study didn't include any information on firearms or other means of suicide, so there isn't any evidence that the two are related. What is interesting is that in other areas the findings mirrored those in the United States in that the number of male suicides was four times the number of female suicides, the highest rates were found in people aged 45 to 54 and over 75, and suicide was the second leading cause of death, after accidents, among youths aged 15 to 24.[55]

Canada isn't exempt from gun violence, but the country's firearm-suicide rate is one-sixth that of the United States, says Jooyoung Lee, a professor at the University of Toronto. The reason, he says, is that "buying a gun is like getting a driver's license. You have to apply for a Possession and Acquisition License—a process that involves a variety of background checks with a minimum 28-day waiting period for new applicants who do not have a valid firearms license." That isn't all. "You have to take a training course. You have to provide personal references who can vouch for your character. You have to renew the license every five years or else you can be charged with unauthorized possession under the Firearms Act and Criminal Code."[56]

The political debate about guns in the United States has focused primarily on universal background checks, a ban on assault weapons, and limits on magazine sizes. In terms of suicide prevention, only the first will have any impact since few people kill themselves with multi-fire AK-47s.

More relevant are laws that require gun owners to lock up their weapons when not in use. Many, especially hunters, gun collectors, and hobbyists, do this already, but others do not. Obviously, if the main reason a person owns a gun is for personal protection, the time required to retrieve it from a locked case might seem to defeat the purpose. Even so, the need to grab a loaded firearm in an instant is rare. Most people are never confronted by a sudden and immediate threat. More often than not, guns are displayed to scare others away.

Storing ammunition separately reduces the risk of an accidental discharge and also lessens the likelihood that a member of the household who may be contemplating suicide can easily access lethal means. This recommendation is endorsed by the American Medical Association, whose journal, *JAMA*, reported that in households with guns, safety procedures like employing gun locks and properly securing ammunition reduce the risk of suicide by two-thirds.[57]

Further evidence is provided by Massachusetts, where youths are 55 percent less likely to die by suicide than youths in other states. The reason? Massachusetts is the only state in the United States that requires residents to lock up guns. Nearly 40 percent of youth suicides nationwide involve a gun, but in Massachusetts guns are used in only 9 percent of youth suicides.[58] (According to the Centers for Disease Control and Prevention, guns were the cause of death in 3.4 of every 100,000 deaths in Massachusetts in 2017, compared with 21.3 per 100,00 in Louisiana and 23.3 per 100,000 in Alaska.)[59]

Another positive step is to encourage health care providers who treat suicidal individuals to ask patients if they have a gun in their house. If the answer is yes, then the next step is to discuss how to keep it away from the person, such as giving it temporarily to someone outside the house, locking it up, or making sure that ammunition isn't stored with it. Forcibly confiscating the gun isn't advised unless the person is delusional and having a gun nearby is dangerous.

"You want to bring about safety through conversation," says Catherine Barber, who directs Harvard's "Means Matter" campaign. "Very rarely do you want to take control away from a person at risk of suicide."[60] Still, even asking the question isn't always possible. A 2011 Center for a New American Security policy brief notes that the National Defense Authorization Act prohibits people in the military from "collecting or recording any information relating to the otherwise lawful acquisition, possession, ownership, carrying, or other use of a privately-owned firearm, privately-owned ammunition, or another private-owned weapon by a member of the Armed Forces" unless the person lives on a military base.[61] In other words, doctors both inside and outside the military can't ask troops who live off base whether they have a gun at home.

The situation is much the same for veterans. In 2020 the Commander John Scott Hannon Veterans Mental Health Care Improvement Act was signed into law. Named in honor of a Navy SEAL who advocated for veterans' mental health treatment before killing himself with a gun in 2018, the act funds community organizations that work with veterans and provides scholarships to train more mental health professionals. A key provision in the act was removed from the bill for political reasons, however, even though it might have saved Hennon's life. It required health care workers who treat veterans to be trained in talking with at-risk patients about the dangers of having guns in the house and how to reduce that risk.[62]

Guns versus Bullets

The comedian Chris Rock once advocated, half jokingly, that there be a hefty tax on bullets to discourage their purchase and use. People laughed at the idea, but there is merit to it. Before he died in 2003, New York senator Daniel Patrick Moynihan said that given the prevalence of guns in this country, it wasn't realistic to think that any federal legislation, even if approved, would make a meaningful difference in controlling gun violence. Anyone who wanted a gun could still get one easily, legally or illegally. A better solution was to tax ammunition. "Guns don't kill people," Moynihan said. "Bullets do."[63]

In 2009 the US Treasury Department reported that in the previous year individuals had bought more than 12 billion rounds of ammunition,[64] equivalent to forty bullets for each gun in the country. In all likelihood, that number is even greater today. Most bullets are used in hunting and target practice, but many gun owners aren't hunters and don't go to gun ranges. They just store bullets in case they ever need to use their guns. At about 50¢ each, bullets are cheap. Moynihan suggested that the police, the military, and perhaps gun ranges could buy bullets tax-free but everyone else would pay a 10,000 percent markup, making the cost $75 per bullet. In addition, the most destructive ammunition, designed for assault weapons and with the ability to pierce armor, would be taxed at an even higher rate.

Taxing bullets might seem unlikely to have much impact on suicides since few suicidal people would be deterred by the cost of a bullet. Where it could make a difference, however, is in reducing the number of bullets that gun owners have. If bullets cost $75 each, there would be less incentive for people to keep a lot of ammunition around. Moreover, accumulating a large number of bullets for the purpose of a mass shooting would be expensive. Four hundred rounds of ammunition, for instance, would cost $30,000.

Gun Reform, Not Gun Control

The key when talking with hunting groups, shooting clubs, and gun-rights groups about reducing gun suicides, says Madeline Drexler, editor of *Harvard Public Health*, a publication of the university's T. H. Chan School of Public Health, isn't to ask, "What do you think of gun control?," because everyone is either for or against it and entrenched in their opinion. The question to ask instead is, "How do we solve the problem of gun suicide?"[65]

John Draper, at one time director of the National Suicide Prevention Lifeline (now the 988 Suicide and Crisis Lifeline), said the same thing in a slightly different way. "If we don't respect that owning a gun is something important to them, individuals, families, and entire communities will stop listening to us altogether. Suicide prevention begins with meeting people where they are, with empathy and respect our greatest tool. If we thought laws were the best answer to preventing suicide, we might seek to make suicides unlawful (again). Until we can legislate a less violent society, out best approach is starting with what we do best . . . listen."[66]

Over a five-day period in 2009, three people who didn't know one another purchased handguns from the same small store in New Hampshire and, within hours, used them to kill themselves. That horrified the store's owner and sent ripples through the community. Rather than being unusual, however, the experience was supported by a study showing that nearly one in ten firearm suicides in New Hampshire involved a gun that had been bought or rented the previous week, often just a few hours before the suicide.[67]

As a result of those deaths, the New Hampshire Gun Shop Project was formed. It was a coalition of mental health professionals, firearm dealers, and gun-rights advocates who banded together to prevent firearm suicides. Posters were created for gun shops to display that listed suicide warning signs and the national Lifeline number. Customers who weren't familiar with firearms were encouraged to get training before they bought a gun and definitely before they used it. Perhaps most important of all, gun dealers were told that they weren't under any obligation to sell someone a gun, particularly if that person looked uneasy or wanted only a small amount of ammunition.

The idea spread quickly, first to Maryland, then to Colorado, and ultimately to at least ten other states. Each state adapted the model to fit its political reality. In Utah, which has one of the highest rates of suicide in the country, the group developed public service announcements that aimed to temporarily separate a potentially suicidal person from his or her gun. *Scientific American*, in a 2017–18 special-issue story on guns and gun violence, compared the approach with the slogan "Friends don't let friends drive drunk." If you are worried about someone's safety, the magazine said, it's your responsibility to take charge and make decisions that the person is incapable of making because their judgment is impaired.

"Go over to their house," said the head of Utah's Shooting Sports Council, "put your arm around them, and say, 'Let me babysit your guns for a while.'" [68]

"What I'm hoping," says one doctor and longtime gun owner, "is that if I ever got into a mess that gloomy, I would remember the poster at the store. I'd remember my training. I would remember that someone once said to me that pointing this thing at yourself is the worst misuse of a gun that could ever be made." [69]

A list of gun safety rules includes an eleventh commandment: that gun owners consider off-site storage of their weapons if a family member is potentially suicidal. Family, friends, shooting clubs, gun shops, and police departments are offered as options. Many gun owners have been receptive to the message. They, as much as any-one, want guns to be used responsibly. One thing they don't want, though, is to be told to stop owning guns. For this reason, when talking about curbing the proliferation of firearms in order to re-duce the number of firearm-related suicides it is important to frame it as "gun reform," not "gun control." This is more than a matter of semantics. "Gun control" is perceived as limiting gun ownership, while the focus of "gun reform" is to make sure that measures are in place so that people who have guns use them responsibly.

The Nature of Alliances

As much as it makes sense for suicide prevention advocates to talk with gun owners, some people believe that there are dangers if they become too close. Tom Zoellner, who wrote a book about the 2011 shooting of Congresswoman Gabby Giffords (who survived but is disabled), has written more recently that the mission of one of the foremost suicide prevention agencies in the country was compro-mised by its association with a gun group.

In 2016 the American Foundation for Suicide Prevention announced a new partnership with the National Sports Shooting

Foundation, which represents thirteen thousand gun dealers and shooting ranges. The goal of the partnership—to reduce the misuse of firearms through various educational campaigns targeted to gun owners—"on the surface seems like a good thing," Zoellner wrote, "a rare example of a gun lobbying group acknowledging a public health problem with its products." But the practical effect, he said, was "to muzzle" the American Foundation for Suicide Prevention from speaking out about gun reform or associating with groups like the Brady Campaign and Women Against Gun Violence.[70]

This concern was reiterated by a former AFSP volunteer whose father had killed himself with a gun he took from a friend's bedroom. In an opinion piece in the *New York Times*, Erin Dunkerly said that after the partnership was announced, volunteers like her "had to keep quiet about gun control." In addition, AFSP "Out of the Darkness" walks like the one Dunkerly chaired in Pasadena were told to exclude gun violence prevention groups that the AFSP deemed to be "interested in gun control."[71]

According to the AFSP, the decision to partner with what it calls "the leading trade association for the firearms industry"[72] was influenced by Harvard's "Means Matter" campaign. That campaign supports engaging with the firearms-owning community for the purpose of reducing gun-related suicides. "Far from being silenced in talking about this issue," Robert Gebbia, CEO of the AFSP, wrote in a letter to the editor following Dunkerly's op-ed, "we are elevating the conversation. . . . Our goal is simple: If you own a gun, we want to bring education about preventing suicide into your community and home." He noted that efforts to reduce gun suicides "have largely failed" and "we must try something new."[73]

When I asked AFSP staff whether "something new" included forbidding chapters from partnering with gun reform groups or instructing volunteers not to discuss or disseminate any information on gun suicides until it was officially approved, the answer was no. According to a spokesperson, the AFSP has cosponsored community events with Everytown for Gun Safety and Moms Demand Action, has been part of an advisory group for the Brady Campaign's public service messaging, and permits any group to set up a table and distribute literature at local AFSP walks as long as they distribute information "related to suicide prevention."

Whether the partnership between the AFSP and the gun industry ultimately is successful depends on how committed the owners of gun shops and shooting ranges are to spreading the message of firearm safety relative to suicide prevention. If they become informed, talk it up regularly, post signs everywhere, reach out to individuals who exhibit suicidal tendencies, and combat the stigma of suicide, which prevents people from seeking help, then the partnership has a good chance of succeeding. At best, it will result in a noticeable drop in firearm suicides. Unfortunately, this hasn't happened yet. More than seven years into the project, the number of gun-related suicides is higher than ever.

Smart Guns

In recent years, so-called smart guns have been developed with built-in safety features that allow only authorized users to fire them. Depending on the manufacturer, there are various ways for these guns to distinguish between authorized and unauthorized users, including fingerprint recognition, radio frequency identification chips, proximity tokens, and mechanical locks. Gun owners have been slow to embrace them, however, because they don't like the idea of having to rely on electronics in situations that they perceive to be potentially life-threatening.

More importantly, the NRA has adamantly opposed "smart guns," going so far as to denounce Smith & Wesson in 2000, when the company came to an agreement with the Clinton administration to develop one. The NRA said that Smith & Wesson was "the first gunmaker to run up the white flag of surrender," released the

CEO's private phone number, and urged its members to voice their complaints. Numerous death threats were received by Smith & Wesson executives, followed by an NRA-led boycott of the company that resulted in a 95 percent drop in the company's stock over the next ten months and the temporary closure of two factories.

"It almost took down the company," said the CEO at the time. "We won't make that mistake again."[73] How well he and other gun manufacturers are able to sleep at night in the wake of so much gun-related violence in this country is something most of us will never know. We do know, though, that in the nineteenth century Sarah Winchester, whose family made the Winchester rifle, was haunted by the ghosts of people killed by it. They drove her to build a half-crazed mansion in the heart of Silicon Valley, but not to cease arms manufacturing.[74]

So where does all this leave us? Do we continue to accept an increasing number of firearm suicides, random gun deaths, and mass shootings as the cost of living—and dying—in America?

In the final chapter I note several steps that can be taken to greatly reduce gun violence in this country, particularly as it relates to gun suicides. These include universal background checks; a ten-day waiting period before purchase of a firearm; "red flag laws," which enable police and immediate family members to remove guns from people who pose a threat to themselves or to others; requiring gunowners to store their weapons safely; and a ban on the sale of high-caliber assault weapons.

None of these take away the existing weapons of responsible gun owners or prevent them from buying more handguns and rifles. None infringe on their rights to protect themselves, to hunt, or to shoot recreationally. Their purpose is to ensure that firearms are used safely, just as traffic codes exist so that drivers operate motor vehicles safely. Is that too much to ask?

CHAPTER 7

Drugs and Suicide

ONE OF THE FEW THINGS ABOUT SUICIDE THAT MANY PEOPLE KNOW, or at least have heard of, isn't a fact but a poem by Dorothy Parker:

> Razors pain you,
> rivers are damp,
> acids stain you,
> and drugs cause cramp.
> Guns aren't lawful,
> nooses give,
> gas smells awful.
> You might as well live.[1]

Like much of Parker's writing, it's acerbic, satirical, and rooted in personal experience—she made three suicide attempts, surviving all three. One can quibble with her statement about guns, which are far from illegal in this country, but her conclusion about choosing life over various means of death (she died at age 73 of a heart attack) is at the center of suicide prevention.

In *Final Exit: The Practicalities of Self-Deliverance and Assisted Suicide for the Dying*, Derek Humphrey lists in similar fashion numerous methods of suicide and the problems with each one. Shooting yourself, he says, is "messy." Hanging is "ugly and extremely traumatic for your loved ones." Carbon monoxide poisoning isn't advised because it has "a high chance of discovery." As for eating poisonous plants, that is "risky and painful," while consuming household chemicals is "painful in the extreme," and cyanide is "difficult to secure." There is always self-starvation, but that isn't "as easy as it sounds." Electrocution is an option but isn't advised "unless you are an ingenious and accomplished electrician."[2]

Humphrey, who founded the Hemlock Society, named after the poison Socrates took to kill himself, came to a different conclusion than Parker. When his first wife at age 40 was diagnosed with cancer, which rapidly consumed her, Humphrey secured, at her request, a lethal dose of Seconal and codeine and gave it to her. Following her death, he became a champion of assisted suicide, and he considered barbiturates "the drug of choice in self-deliverance."[3]

Today, drugs are the means of choice for 70 percent of people who attempt suicide. This includes over-the-counter medication like Tylenol and prescription pills like Seconal. It also includes painkillers like fentanyl and oxycodone, as well as illegal opiates like heroin, although these drugs, while responsible for many deaths, often result in overdoses that are considered accidental rather than intentional.

If a young woman swallows a bottle full of sleeping pills, her intention is fairly obvious, but if she dies with a needle in her arm, it's uncertain whether she wanted to kill herself. If a man chases pills with alcohol, there is a good chance that his death is a suicide, but if he snorts white-powder heroin that has been cut with fentanyl or even baking soda and then dies, a strong argument can be made that it was an accident. Unless a coroner is certain, it won't be ruled a suicide until more information, such as a suicide note, is found. That might not happen, especially if family members don't want it to.

The relationship between drugs and suicide is further complicated by the fact that drugs are both a means of suicide and a risk factor for it. They are a means because they offer the seemingly peaceful prospect of falling asleep and never waking up. People may not have access to a gun, know how to direct their car's exhaust, be willing to hang themselves, or want to jump from a high place, but swallowing a bunch of pills is easy and seemingly painless. Drugs are a risk factor for suicide because people who are under the influence of drugs or alcohol tend to lose their inhibitions and take risks that they normally wouldn't take. Also, sedatives and depressants like alcohol can bring on symptoms of depression.

"As the consequences of addiction pile up," wrote Dr. Carolyn Ross in *Psychology Today*, "from legal problems and damaged relationships to financial ruin and job loss, individuals may lose all hope that things can get better. For some, it starts to seem like there are only two paths to relief; spiraling back into drug use or death."[4] There is a third path, to try and stop using, but that can have negative consequences too. Stopping can mean that painful emotions that drugs have pushed down return in force, leaving a person vulnerable and depressed. Alternatively, the person might be clearheaded enough to act on suicidal thoughts and plans.

The bottom line is that people who are dependent on drugs or alcohol are five times as likely to attempt suicide as the general population. For women, a substance abuse disorder increases the risk of suicide by six and a half times.[5]

A Growing Epidemic

In 2018 there were 68,000 overdose deaths in the United States—a record.[6] In 2019 the number was 71,000—a new record.[7] In 2020 it was 93,000, a 29 percent increase.[8] The number rose again in 2021, to 107,000.[9] Some experts attributed the increase to the pandemic because treatment was hard to get then and many people living on the edge had more money than usual because evictions were suspended and unemployment benefits were extended. That failed to explain why the number went up again in 2022, however, to a new high of nearly 110,000.[10]

For over-the-counter medications, no one has to go far. They are available at any pharmacy and many supermarkets around the country with no restrictions. People who shop at big discount stores are spared the inconvenience of buying numerous small packages. Costco, for instance, sells 500 mg tablets of extra-strength acetaminophen (the generic form of Tylenol) in containers of 1,000 capsules.

Even for sedatives like Seconal, which usually require a prescription, procurement s fairly straightforward. A person merely has to complain to a physician that they are suffering from insomnia or anxiety. A large segment of the population suffers from these afflictions, yet this suffering is hard to prove, so most physicians have no choice but to accept a patient's word for it.

It's not that way in some other countries. In England, for instance, legislation passed in 1998 limits the pack size of analgesics and prohibits pharmacies from selling more than thirty-two tablets to a single customer (other sellers are restricted from selling more than sixteen tablets per customer). In 2004 the *British Medical Journal* reported that after the legislation was implemented in England, there was a 22 percent decrease in the number of suicides related to acetaminophen overdoses and a 30 percent decrease in the number of liver transplants and in the number of admissions to hospital liver units (overdosing on acetaminophen severely damages the liver).[11] Similarly, suicides in Australia from sedative overdoses were fairly common when these medications were easy to obtain but decreased when access was restricted.[12]

There are several ways to restrict access to medications. The first is to reduce the pack size. The second is to limit the number of packs a person can buy at any one time. The third is to require blister tabs on medications that are harmful if consumed in larger quantities than recommended. A blister tab is special packaging that requires a person to press a tab, usually with the thumb or forefinger, to dispense a pill. Only one pill can be dispensed at a time, and if one presses the tab continually in order to get more pills, one is likely to incur a blister. That might seem inconsequential when a person intends to swallow a large handful of pills at once; however, any kind of deterrent is effective in reducing suicide. The mere fact that it takes a while to accumulate a sufficient number can discourage people from resorting to that means or cause them to eject fewer pills than needed to kill themselves, making intervention possible.

"Twenty or 30 years ago," writes George Howe Colt, "depressed and possibly self-destructive people were likely to be treated with psychotherapy, supported, where indicated, by medication. By the new millennium, drugs were the treatment of choice—in most cases the only treatment—for depression as well as nearly every other psychiatric condition."[13] Cost was the main reason for the change; drugs are cheaper than psychotherapy. They are also more convenient for consumers. Instead of driving to a therapist's office and talking for fifty minutes, a person can just go to the medicine cabinet.

Colt goes on to say, "These days, few clinicians would suggest that psychotherapy alone, without medication to address the underlying illness, is enough to prevent profoundly suicidal individuals from killing themselves. Yet many would maintain that medication alone is enough to deal with depressed and typically suicidal individuals."[14] This is especially true in the military, where active-duty service members and veterans routinely are prescribed pills of all kinds to deal with PTSD and other psychological issues in lieu of counseling. If one kind of pill doesn't solve the problem, other kinds of pills—or multiple pills—are prescribed.

Among the most frequently prescribed pills are selective serotonin reuptake inhibitors, commonly referred to as SSRIs, used to treat depression, aggressive behavior, and impulsivity, and to this end they have been effective. They are enormously popular, with name brands like Prozac and Zoloft accounting for billions of dollars in worldwide sales every year. The problem is that relieving symptoms of psychiatric illness isn't the same thing as dealing with root causes. Moreover, there is evidence suggesting that antidepressants have the adverse effect of increasing the risk of suicide among young people. In 2004, after dozens of parents alleged that the drugs had contributed to their children's death, the makers were required to include warnings on labels that a potential consequence was an elevated risk "of suicidal thinking and behavior in children and teens."[15]

Opioids

Opioids include both prescription painkillers and illegal drugs like heroin, which can become addictive. Some common prescription opioids and their commercial names are oxycodone (OxyContin, Percocet), hydrocodone (Vicodin), meperidine (Dolophine), and morphine (Roxanol).

According to a 2017 study in the *American Journal of Public Health*, the number of suicides involving opioids more than doubled between 1999 and 2014. That increase was less than the increase in the number of opioid deaths overall, the majority of which were accidental, but it still represented a growth in opioid suicides nationwide from 2 percent to 4 percent. The increase was greater for women than for men, for whites than for other ethnicities, and for middle-aged Americans than for younger people. Perhaps most surprising, nearly 98 percent of opioid-related suicides involved prescription painkillers, while only .03 percent involved heroin (a naturally derived opiate). The authors of the study, which was led by researchers at the University of Washington, noted that most of the suicides were by people with histories of depression and PTSD, who tended to be prescribed higher doses for longer periods of time than the general population.[16]

At the time when the study was released, the opioid epidemic had become so bad that *CNN* aired a story on librarians who were learning to treat overdoses. One librarian, ten years out of college and working in Philadelphia, saved six people in a single month. Her library was next to a small park, and heroin users shot up in the library's bathroom. By injecting the drug Narcan to reverse the effect of an overdose, the librarian, whose parents had used heroin, revived unconscious addicts and watched them until medical help arrived.[17]

Also in 2017 Dr. Maria Oquendo, president of the American Psychiatric Association, briefed Congress on opioid use. She said that research had shown that men with opioid use disorder (OUD) were twice as likely to die by suicide as men without the disorder, and women with OUD were eight times as likely to kill themselves as other women. While the national suicide rate at the time was 14 per 100,000 people, the suicide rate of people with OUD was 87 per 100,000, with the highest increase among those aged 45 to 64.[18]

In a subsequent article in the *New England Journal of Medicine*, Oquendo referenced the difficulty of separating voluntary overdose deaths from unintentional ones before noting that about 15 percent of the 45,000 suicides in 2016 in the United States had been drug overdoses. More telling were the results from the Nationwide Emergency Department Sample of 250,000-plus emergency department visits by adults for an opiate overdose. Nearly 27 percent were deemed intentional.[19]

A 2017 study published in the *Journal of Psychiatric Research* concluded that the misuse of prescription opioids was associated with a 40–60 percent increase in suicide ideation. Moreover, individuals who routinely exceeded the prescribed dosage were 75 percent more likely to plan their suicides and two times more likely to make an attempt.[20]

OxyContin, the number-one prescribed painkiller for many years, was first marketed in 1996 and quickly became the top brand-name narcotic pain reliever. In places like West Virginia and Kentucky it replaced moonshine as the drug of choice, to the extent that it became known as "hillbilly heroin."[21] Prescriptions were easy to obtain, no preparation was required, and the buzz was euphoric, or at least numbing, as with heroin. Oxy is far from cheap, however. The street price is $1 per milligram, and it's not unusual for addicts to need 400 to 500 milligrams a day.[22] By contrast, the going rate for a small balloon with one dose of heroin is $9, and heavy users consume ten doses a day.[23] That's $90 compared with $500. *Per day.* Given the economics, it's no wonder that four out of five heroin addicts say that they transitioned to smack from prescription painkillers.[24]

In 2019, when the CDC reported 71,000 overdose deaths in the United States—nearly 5 percent more than in 2018—the greatest increase was in South Dakota (54 percent), followed by North Dakota (31 percent), and Alaska (27 percent).[25] A year later, experts feared that the numbers would be even worse, exacerbated by the coronavirus, and they were right. Overdose deaths rose to 93,655, with more than half from fentanyl, oxycodone, and other synthetic opioids. In 2021 they increased again, to 107,622, with nearly 70 percent attributable to fentanyl and related drugs.[26] The same was true in 2022, when more than 75 percent of the 109,680 overdose deaths were the result of opioids.[27]

The CDC doesn't distinguish between accidental drug overdoses and suicides, but another 2019 CDC report notes a significant and continuing trend. Historically, drug overdose deaths have been higher in Appalachia and other rural areas, but now they are slightly higher in cities (22 deaths per 100,000 people compared with 20 deaths per 100,000 people in rural areas). The CDC attributes the change to an increase in illegal drugs like heroin, for which the distribution system is more developed in cities, and to greater heroin use in affluent suburban areas by whites.[28]

There are multiple reasons why transitioning from Oxy to heroin is dangerous. One is that heroin often is cut, so users don't know what they are getting. Second, heroin frequently is injected, and users may not handle needles safely. Third, the immediate effect differs depending on how it's consumed. A person who snorts heroin has to inhale twice as much to achieve the same rush as through injection, and there is a lag time of about ten minutes before the euphoria hits after snorting, whereas injection produces an immediate high. The danger with snorting is that inexperienced users don't know how much they have consumed, and if they don't think anything is happening, they continue to inhale until the effect is lethal. This makes heroin far riskier than OxyContin, although OxyContin is risky enough.

Most people consume opioids not with the intention of killing themselves but because they want to get high or to dull their physical pain. It's only after they become addicted that the dynamics change. As one user told Beth Macy, author of *Dopesick: Dealers, Doctors, and the Drug Company That Addicted America*, "At the end of your journey, you're not doing it to get high; you're doing it to keep from being dope sick."[29] *Dope sick* refers to the illness following the withdrawal of heroin or other opiates, and Macy says that there are more than two million people with OUD in the United States. Others put the number slightly lower, while others believe it's higher. Either way, the opioid crisis has reached epidemic proportions in this country.

One bright spot is that in recent years governmental agencies have been cracking down on so-called pill mills, where doctors over-prescribe OxyContin, Vicodin, Percocet, and other painkillers. The practice was especially egregious in Florida, but after doctors there were barred from selling drugs that they prescribed, deaths from narcotic pain relievers dropped by 26 percent.[30] Today, many states have databases that track prescriptions of addictive painkillers so that physicians can see whether patients are "doctor shopping" and getting pills at multiple locations. In addition, a growing number of physicians are facing criminal charges for writing excessive prescriptions of OxyContin that result in overdose deaths, which is having a positive impact in terms of discouraging the practice.

Another bright spot is that Purdue Pharma, the Connecticut-based company that manufactured OxyContin and maintained for years that the drug wasn't addictive, admitted under growing pressure that it was. A multi-billion-dollar settlement was negotiated, and the Sackler family, which owned the company, was forced to relinquish control.

A third bright spot is that in recent years the number of doctors certified to prescribe Suboxone has more than doubled, according to reporting by the *New York Times*.[31] Suboxone, which dissolves under the tongue, is the brand name of buprenorphine, which keeps drug users from experiencing cravings and withdrawal, making it easier for them to move off heroin and other opioids.

The irony, in case anyone misses it, is that the industry that created the problem and has made billions of dollars off it is now creating a slew of drugs to treat it, making billions of dollars more. Three of the main companies that manufacture naloxone products (of which Narcan is a specific brand) increased their prices by at least 500 percent over a nine-year period as demand for the drug increased. Indivior, which makes Suboxone, signed a seven-year licensing agreement with the Food and Drug Administration to sell its product free of competition, enabling it to charge whatever it wants. Two of the companies that make a different class of drugs, ones that are used to treat opioid-induced constipation, doubled their price from $173 in 2007 to $350 in 2017, while a third company selling the same kind of drug charges $1,500.[32]

After aggressively marketing opioids for years as a low-risk solution for chronic and severe pain, pharmaceutical companies have been more than willing to help people get off them—for a price. At the same time, the industry continues to push opioid use, both in the United States and abroad. In fact, overseas markets are providing new opportunities. In Australia, for instance, opioid-related deaths doubled from 2006 to 2016, most of them from OxyContin and other prescription drugs rather than illegal opioids like heroin.[33]

Not that heroin has always been illegal. As Erin Marie Daly notes in *Generation Rx: A Story of Dope, Death, and America's Opiate Crisis*, at one time the Bayer Company sold heroin over the counter in the United States, in both pill and elixir forms, as a cough suppressant. The company claimed that the risk of addiction was low; however, there was "an explosion of heroin-relation admissions at hospitals," Daly writes, with many users supporting their habit by collecting and selling scrap metal. Thus, the origination of the term *junkie*.[34]

Inasmuch as Big Pharma is nearly as powerful as the National Rifle Association, there is resistance when it comes to cracking down on pill mills and forcing physicians to cut back on prescriptions of highly addictive painkillers. Nevertheless, both efforts have social and political support, especially as the number of overdose deaths keeps rising. Requiring companies to package certain over-the-counter medications with blister tabs and in smaller amounts might seem more challenging, but it doesn't have to be. Companies will pass the cost along to consumers, just as they do when they are required to make products tamper-proof, or as car manufacturers do when they add airbags, blind-spot warning systems, backup cameras, and other safety features to their vehicles. As a result, companies won't be out anything.

Consumers, in turn, probably won't notice that their medication costs a few cents more than it used to, or if they do notice, they will attribute the added cost to corporate markup, not to any packaging change. Moreover, if smaller quantities and blister tabs become the norm, consumers will accept it because they won't have a choice. The only real change will be that some medications can't be abused as easily. To my mind, that matters more than anything else.

CHAPTER 8

Jump Sites and Suicide

THERE IS A MAJOR DIFFERENCE BETWEEN FALLS AND JUMPS. Getting too close to the edge of a cliff or a tall structure and unintentionally going over the side is different from leaping from the spot intentionally. The distinction is important because the public reacts to falls and jumps quite differently. Falls are accidents and could happen to anyone who isn't careful, while jumps are suicides and generally of little concern to individuals who have no desire to die. As a result, most people support measures to protect against falls, such as guardrails on mountain roads and fences around swimming pools, but argue over anything that makes a potential jump site safer, such as a tall railing or a net.

In the United States, jump sites—bridges, tall buildings, cliffs, freeway overpasses, and train crossings—account for about 5 percent of suicides, or more than two thousand per year.[1] That's a small number compared with the number of people who kill themselves with a firearm, although it's by no means insignificant. In some other countries, notably England and Australia, where cliffs are popular jumps sites, and Japan, where there has been a rash of suicides from the windows and rooftops of office buildings, jumping to one's death is common.

The attraction of jump sites is twofold. First, death is virtually guaranteed. It's almost impossible to survive a fall of more than one hundred feet, especially if the person lands on pavement, rocks, or other hard ground. Second, death is immediate. There is no more than a split second of pain before the end comes. A third, less important reason is that no work is required beyond getting to the site. One doesn't need to acquire anything, learn anything, or do anything. One just needs to get to the site and jump. An added benefit in the minds of some suicidal people, particularly those who jump from bridges, is that either the person goes under and disappears forever or their body is recovered by strangers, often Coast Guard crew members or boaters. Either way, loved ones are spared a gruesome sight.

Bridges

In 2008 the National Suicide Prevention Lifeline, based in New York City and operating the nation's primary suicide hotline (formerly 800-283-TALK; now 988), issued a position paper approved by the steering committee, on which I served. The paper concluded that installing physical barriers on bridges was the most effective way to prevent bridge suicides. Other measures, such as signage and phones, increased awareness and were "a supplement to bridge barriers" but not an end in themselves.[2]

The Lifeline paper, which was revised and updated in 2017, was issued after the New York State Bridge Authority installed phones on five bridges in the Catskill region of the state, as well as signs that encouraged anyone who was suicidal to call the Lifeline's toll-free number. The bridge authority cited issues pertaining to weight, wind, snow, and safety inspection as reasons why physical barriers couldn't be erected on any of the bridges and hailed the program as a "model for other bridge authorities around the nation"[3] despite the lack of any evidence regarding its effectiveness.

Afterward, opponents of barriers on bridges in Ithaca, New York, and Santa Barbara, California, used the New York State Bridge Authority's report to support their claim that phones and signs were sufficient to stop suicides. Anything more, such as barriers, wasn't needed, they said. This was music to the ears of many officials because phones and signs are cheap compared with barriers. Also, calls are answered by another entity, usually the Lifeline's national network of affiliated crisis centers, so there isn't any other cost. This was what prompted the Lifeline to take a formal position on the issue.

"Bridge or transportation authorities may choose to install bridge phones linked to local suicide prevention call centers as cost-saving mechanisms over installing bridge barriers," the Lifeline paper said; however, "Lifeline is unable to recommend this approach as the first, most effective, empirically-validated course of action in preventing suicides from bridges."[4] The updated Lifeline paper notes that two years after phones were installed on five bridges in New York, eleven people jumped to their death including six from the Newburgh-Beacon Bridge. In addition, suicide hotline phones and related signage were installed on other bridges around the country with no verifiable effect. This included the top four bridges in the United States in terms of suicide jumps—the Golden Gate Bridge in San Francisco, Aurora Bridge in Seattle, Coronado Bay Bridge in San Diego, and Sunshine Skyway Bridge in St. Petersburg, Florida.[5]

Crisis line phones were first installed on the Golden Gate Bridge in 1993. Since then, at least one thousand people have jumped from the bridge, and there is no evidence that any of them tried to call beforehand. The simple fact is that suicidal people are in too much of a daze to notice the phones or to care. Obviously, it doesn't help that there are numerous photos on the internet of crisis phones on the Golden Gate Bridge with "Out or Order" signs.

The Golden Gate Bridge has an added element that most other bridges don't have: surveillance equipment. More than fifty cameras, both above the roadway and underneath the span, monitor vehicle traffic and pedestrian activity. For years, Golden Gate Bridge District officials touted this equipment as part of their suicide-prevention efforts even though it wasn't installed with that purpose in mind. Rather, as an international landmark, the bridge is thought to be a potential target for terrorists, and the equipment is in place to identify a possible terrorist attack. It was beefed up substantially after 9/11, and today security police man a control room 24 hours a day, 365 days a year, watching TV monitors. The images are live—looking down on traffic, following pedestrians and bicyclists, monitoring the toll plaza—and officers can change the views in an instant to show any section of the bridge, then zoom in. Lights on the bridge make it possible to view camera images after nightfall, although heavy fog sometimes obscures visibility. Next to the control room is a smaller room that has additional monitors and recording equipment. This is where officers go to rewind and review surveillance tapes.

Seattle's Aurora Bridge was the second deadliest bridge in the United States after the Golden Gate Bridge with more than four hundred suicides. Emergency call boxes and signs were installed in 2006, but until 2011 five people per year on average jumped from the bridge. That was the year when fencing was installed. In the following year there was only one suicide from the bridge.[6]

Surveillance equipment, suicide hotline phones, and signs proclaiming "Life is worth living" haven't had much effect on suicides from New York City's Verrazzano-Narrows Bridge. Three people jumped to their death from the bridge within one month in 2019, prompting a Brooklyn councilman to make an impassioned plea to fellow council members. He said that his heart broke every time he heard helicopters in the middle of the night or early morning because it meant that another person had jumped and the bridge needed a barrier.[7] At the time of this writing, his proposal hasn't been acted on.

In San Diego, phones and signs haven't reduced the number of suicides from the Coronado Bay Bridge, which opened in 1969, is three miles long, and has been the site of more than four hundred suicides to date. A suicide barrier has been discussed but remains years away. In response to community and political pressure, the California Department of Transportation, referred to colloquially as Caltrans, installed metal spikes on the bridge's railing as a temporary suicide deterrent. The spikes were similar to those that are used to prevent pigeons and other birds from roosting on ledges and roofs. It's clear, however, that the spikes have had no effect. Fifteen people jumped to their death from the Coronado Bridge in 2019 after the spikes were installed, consistent with the average of two to nineteen suicides per year from the bridge. The only effect of the spikes, according to one firefighter, has been that people jump quickly because they can't sit on the railing and contemplate their decision.[8]

Crisis phones were installed on the Sunshine Skyway Bridge in Florida in 1999. Over the next three years, twenty-two people jumped to their death from the bridge.[9] In 2018, eighteen people died by jumping from the bridge, and the installation of fencing was approved in 2020 and installed in June 2021. A year later, in June 2022, four people still managed to jump and die.[10]

"While it may be true that suicide hotline call boxes on 'suicide-prone bridges' have successfully prevented suicide for individuals who have chosen to use them," the Lifeline paper states, "it is also clear that many suicides have occurred from bridges where they have been present. Placing a hotline phone on a bridge provides a 'rescue option' for suicidal individuals who are knowingly ambivalent. However, for other persons who come to the bridge that are consumed with psychological pain and intent on dying, relying on them to pick up the phone and call in that climactic moment places too much confidence in their capacity to still make a rational choice." This is why it's hard to argue against the efficacy of bridge barriers. At numerous sites around the world that once were suicide magnets, a barrier has ended, or virtually ended, the problem.

At one time the Bloor Street Bridge in Toronto, also known as the Prince Edward Viaduct, was considered the second deadliest bridge in the world after the Golden Gate Bridge, with 480 fatal jumps. Then in 2003 the city spent $4 million on a "luminous veil" of ten thousand stainless steel rods. The rods are so thin that one person compared them to the strings on a Stradivarius violin, yet they create an impenetrable wall. The barrier had the desired effect: the number of suicides dropped to zero and has stayed there.[11] Of added interest, the barrier received the Canadian national engineering award for design elegance. Many people thought that the aesthetics of the bridge were enhanced by the barrier, which today is referred to as "lifesaving art." It's worth noting that funding was allocated following the death of a 35-year-old man who jumped from the bridge after walking past toll-free phones connected to the city's suicide hotline.[12]

A more dramatic example is the Grafton Bridge in Auckland, New Zealand. Safety barriers were removed from the bridge in 1996 after being in place for sixty years. Officials there thought they weren't needed anymore. Over the next six years there were fifteen suicides from the bridge. When the barriers were reinstalled in 2003, no further suicides occurred, nor was there a "substitution effect," with neighboring bridges experiencing an increase in the number of suicides.[13]

In Bristol, England, a partial barrier was erected on the Clifton Suspension Bridge. Over five years the number of suicides from the bridge was reduced from eight to four. Researchers concluded that there would have been even fewer suicides if a full barrier had been in place. Moreover, they noted that there had been no increase in the number of jumps from other bridges.[14]

A different example is the Swiss town of Bern. Prior to 1998, about 60 percent of suicides in Switzerland's capital city were the result of jumps from tall bridges and other structures. Three or four of these per year were from the Munsterplattform, a famous cathedral with dramatic views. After a net was installed there, suicides ended. Subsequently, the Bern City Parliament voted to install nets on several bridges in the city that had been suicide sites. Bern's success became the model that Golden Gate Bridge District officials cited when they proposed adding a net under the world-famous span.[15]

In the United States, there were fourteen suicides from 1960 to 1983 on Memorial Bridge in Augusta, Maine. After a barrier was installed, the number dropped to zero. Two decades later, a researcher at the Centers for Disease Control and Prevention reported that no other site in the area had registered an increase in suicides; in fact, there had been an overall decrease in the number of suicides in the city. He concluded that the bridge barrier "was probably effective in lowering the overall suicide rate in Augusta."[16]

In 2004, the bridge was due to be renovated, and the question was raised whether the barrier was still needed. After all, twenty years had passed without a single suicide. To their credit, city council members voted to retain it. "Some see that fence as something ugly," one council member told the local paper, "but I see it as something caring. The fence is a symbol that tells motorists and pedestrians that the capital city is concerned about the mentally ill who live here."[17]

From 1979 through 1985, twenty-four people died by jumping off the Duke Ellington Bridge in Washington, DC. In 1986 an eight-foot-high antisuicide fence was constructed following three suicides in a ten-day period. One of the suicides was the 24-year-old daughter of Ben Read, a former deputy secretary of state. Five years after the barrier was installed, only one person had jumped from the bridge. Furthermore, there was no increase in the number of suicides from the nearby Taft Bridge, which didn't have a barrier.

In Pasadena, California, there have been more than 150 suicides from the Colorado Street Bridge since the bridge opened in 1919, so many that locals refer to it as the "Suicide Bridge." One hundred fifty feet above Arroyo Seco, a water-carved canyon, the bridge was especially popular as a suicide site during the Great Depression. In 2017, after a spate of suicide attempts, a temporary chain-link fence the length of the bridge was installed. Only one person has jumped since, and the city council is looking into having a permanent barrier installed. Donald McDonald and Associates, the same firm that helped design the safety net under the Golden Gate Bridge, has been commissioned to design it.[18]

The point is that in every instance in which a physical barrier—a taller railing, fencing, or a net—has been installed at a bridge that once was a popular suicide site, suicides from that bridge have been greatly reduced or ended and there hasn't been an increase in the number of suicides from neighboring bridges or in the number of local suicides by other means. Those are facts.

In 2018 Toronto Public Health issued a comprehensive report, *Interventions to Prevent Suicide from Bridges: An Evidence Review and Jurisdictional Scan*. The report was prompted by 125 suicides from bridges in Toronto from 2004 to 2015, an average of 10 suicides per year. Other bridges in Canada (two in Vancouver and one in Edmonton), as well as bridges outside the country (in England, Switzerland, and the United States, most notably the Golden Gate Bridge), were included in the study. Three types of interventions were identified: restricting access by installing barriers and nets; encouraging help-seeking behaviors by installing phones and signage; and increasing the likelihood of intervention by police, firefighters, or bridge workers through the use of surveillance cameras.

The report covers seven Canadian bridges with barriers (one each in Toronto, Edmonton, Montreal, Surrey, and Halifax and two in Vancouver), eight bridges in the United States with barriers (in Akron, Augusta, Pasadena, Santa Barbara, Seattle, and Washington, DC), seven bridges in the United States with nets (all spanning the city of Ithaca and Cornell University), and fourteen bridges in other countries with barriers (one each in the Czech Republic, Luxembourg, New Zealand, Norway, Scotland, South Africa, Spain, and the United Kingdom, and six in Australia). The report also notes twenty-three bridges in Canada and elsewhere in the world with crisis phones and signage (including fourteen in the United States) and nine bridges with surveillance cameras (four in the United States).[19] "Of these," the report states, "studies have found that means restriction interventions, such as bridge barriers, were associated with a 93 percent reduction in suicide deaths per year when implemented as a sole intervention. More evidence is needed to determine the effectiveness of other interventions."[20]

One site not mentioned in the report, no doubt owing to a lack of available information, was the Nanjing Yangtze River Bridge in China. Nanjing has a population of six million people, many of whom cross the four-mile bridge every day. At least one suicide is said to occur weekly from the bridge, which is 130 feet above the Yangtze River. On an annual basis, that means more suicides than anywhere else in the world, although the bridge still has a long way to go before the total number of suicides rivals that of the Golden Gate Bridge. Signs are posted discouraging suicide, and volunteers patrol the span looking for people who might be thinking of jumping (a short film about one volunteer, *Angel of Nanjing*, can be found on YouTube). At one point the Chinese government smeared butter on the Nanjing bridge's railing, hoping to make it too slippery to surmount. It was a fanciful idea, but like signage it didn't have any effect. Suicides from the bridge continued.

Other Jump Sites

Bridges aren't the only jump sites. Cliffs are popular with some suicidal individuals for the same reason as bridges: they are easily accessible and often unprotected, death is quick and nearly certain, and recovery of the body is left to strangers, if it's recovered at all.

Beachy Head is in many respects quintessential England. As Tom Hunt notes in his book *Cliffs of Despair: A Journey to Suicide's Edge*, green pastures end at a windy promontory that overlooks the sea. Each year, nearly five hundred thousand people visit the site, which is as beautiful as it is deadly. Since 1965 more than five hundred people have walked, jumped, or intentionally driven off the treacherous, unguarded, 535-foot-high cliffs. According to Hunt, at one time Princess Diana allegedly went to Beachy Head intending to jump. Residents refer to the local tavern—where, says Hunt, they whisper among themselves about men and women there who are silent and hollow-eyed and appear to be having a final drink before ending their lives—as the Last Stop Pub. A woman who is celebrated locally as a witch claims that Beachy Head was once the site of human sacrifices.[21]

There are no physical barriers at Beachy Head. About twenty people kill themselves every year there. A small number of casualties at Beachy Head aren't suicides. They are people who have gotten too close to the edge and fallen after a large chunk of cliff broke off. The lower cliffs continue to erode from wave action, which causes pieces of the upper cliffs to crack and eventually collapse into the sea.

The Beachy Head Chaplaincy Team patrols the area day and night in an effort to locate and stop potential jumpers. Pub workers and taxi drivers are on the lookout for possible suicide victims as well. Signs are posted bearing the phone number of the Samaritans, a charitable organization that provides phone support to distressed and suicidal people in the United Kingdom and Ireland, comparable in some ways to the 988 Suicide and Crisis Lifeline in the United States.

In Australia, a rocky cliff at the entrance to Sydney Harbour called The Gap is a notorious suicide site. Some 330 feet above the Pacific Ocean, it is the place where roughly fifty people kill themselves each year by leaping onto rocks or into the water below.[22] For nearly his entire adult life, a man known by locals as "the Angel of The Gap" made it his mission to persuade people not to jump. From 1964 until his death from natural causes in 2012, Don Ritchie watched out for suicidal people from his home across the street. Anytime he saw someone who was alone and standing close to the edge of the precipice, he hurried to their side, smiled, and asked, "Can I help you in some way?" More than once he risked his own life by physically restraining someone, but most of the time his quiet approach had an effect. Afterward, he would invite the person to his home for a cup of tea and further conversation. He never tried to counsel, offer advice, or pry into people's lives; he just listened as a friend and genuinely cared.

Ritchie is described by people who knew him as a modest and humble man who didn't seek accolades or media attention for his work. He was, in his wife's words, "an everyday person who did an extraordinary thing for many people that saved their lives, without any want of recognition."[23]

When asked, Ritchie couldn't remember the first suicide he had witnessed, nor was he haunted by the people he couldn't save. He just did the best job he could, he said, and felt fortunate rather than burdened regarding the location of his home. Ritchie didn't keep count, but he estimated that he had saved more than 160 people over the years. Late in life he told a reporter, "My ambition has always been to just get them away from the edge, to buy them time, to give them the opportunity to reflect and give them the chance to realize that things might look better the next morning. . . . You can't just sit there and watch them. You have to try and save them. It's pretty simple."[24]

While Ritchie was alive, The Gap had a barrier of sorts—a three-foot-high fence. In 2016 the prime minister of Australia announced that the fence would be raised and closed-circuit TV cameras would be installed, along with emergency phones, lighting, and signs, to prevent more suicides. The new fence is concave, making it hard for someone to get a foothold. It's not much higher than the old fence—only four and a quarter feet high—but it's better than what was there. Its main function is to act as a psychological impediment. "We know it is not impossible to climb," said a spokeswoman for the project, "but it's about buying time by making it difficult so that those considering suicide may stop to reconsider."[25] Even an extra minute or two may be all that is needed for bystanders to reach someone intent on jumping and to talk them down.

When a person feels that life is unbearable and suicide is the only way out, barring access to lethal means, such as a gun, drugs, or a jump site, makes all the difference. The *California Strategic Plan on Suicide Prevention*, which I helped draft, notes, "Restricting access to lethal means can put time between the impulse to complete suicide and the act itself, allowing opportunities for the impulse to subside or warning signs to be recognized."[26]

Says Dr. Rebecca Bernert, a psychologist and head of suicide-prevention studies at Stanford University, "What we know about means restriction is that it works. If you put time and space between thoughts regarding suicide and access to means, you save lives."[27]

After a detailed study of "suicide hotspots," including bridges, England's National Institute of Mental Health concluded that "the most effective form of prevention at jumping sites is a physical barrier, which literally restricts access to the drop."[28]

The Lessons of Japan

In 2016 Japan's suicide rate (18.5 per 100,000 people) was the second highest among developed countries, behind only South Korea.[29] Among people aged 15 to 39, suicide is the primary cause of death in Japan, where the number of people who kill themselves is higher than the combined number of those who die from cancer and accidents.[30] Among G-7 countries, Japan is the only one where suicide is the leading manner of death.

Japan has a long history of suicide, dating back to the twelfth century, when samurai engaged in seppuku, disemboweling themselves in a ritual that was intended to avoid the shame and dishonor of failing to protect their lords. The practice continued in World War II, with kamikaze pilots flying into Allied warships. Today, suicide is viewed as a public health crisis in Japan, and there is a focus on more supportive services for people contemplating suicide, such as counseling and suicide hotlines, and also on cultural shifts, such as changes in employment laws that make for shorter work weeks.

As noted previously, it's illegal in Japan for private citizens to own firearms, so the most common method of suicide is hanging. Many of the deaths have occurred in the Aokigahara Forest, also known as the Sea of Trees, at the base of Mount Fuji. The trees grow so close together within the forest's fourteen square miles that they block out the sun and the wind, leaving few animals, birds, or sounds. In addition, bodies can remain undiscovered there for months.

The combination of solitude and privacy makes the Sea of Trees the perfect place to die, according to the *Complete Manual of Suicide*, published in Japan in 1993.[31] At least five hundred people have wandered into the forest, thrown a rope over a low-hanging branch, and hanged themselves. (The actual number is unknown because Japanese authorities don't want to make the forest even more popular with suicidal people.) The bodies are found by volunteers who clean the forest, with many victims being Japanese businessmen who have been affected by economic downturns. Some victims, though, have been drawn there after reading the Japanese novel *Kuroi Jukai*, by Seicho Matsumoto, which ends with a couple's joint suicide in the Aokigahara Forest. Signs posted by police on trees to discourage suicides—"Your life is a precious gift from your parents," "Please consult the police before you decide to die!"—have had little effect. From ten to thirty people are found hanging in the forest each year; some bodies are never found because the trees grow so close together.[32]

Jump sites also are popular among suicidal people in Japan, particularly skyscrapers since the small footprint of the country, combined with its highly concentrated population centers, makes for numerous tall buildings. Access to many rooftops is blocked, but it's still possible for employees to open windows and jump. In a few places, canopies have been strung like a firefighter's net to catch people before they hit the ground, but in Tokyo, in particular, the tall office buildings are too numerous for that to make much difference.

Two other popular jump sites in Japan are public and accessible to everyone. One is Mount Mihara, an active volcano on the island of Izu Oshima. In 1933 a Japanese student made headlines when she jumped into the crater. She was in love with another woman, which was considered taboo at the time, and talked about taking her life in that way long before she did it. Following her death, more than 900 people (804 men and 140 women) also jumped into the volcano. Eventually the deaths subsided, owing partly to increased security and partly to a new rule that made it illegal to buy a one-way ticket to the island.[33]

The other popular jump site is the Tojinbo cliffs, eighty feet above the Sea of Japan. Like Don Ritchie at The Gap in Australia, Yukio Shige has frequented the cliffs as a guardian angel for more than fifteen years. A retired policeman, he and a team of twenty other volunteers claim to have talked more than six hundred suicidal people back from the edge. Shige's approach, like Ritchie's, is simple. "It's not exciting or anything," he says. "I'm like, 'Hey, how are you doing?' These people are asking for help. They're just waiting for someone to speak to them."[34]

Covid-19 has exacerbated the problem. In October 2020 alone, there were more suicides in Japan (2,153) than there were deaths from the pandemic for the entire year (2,087). Women in particular were affected. While male deaths in Japan were 22 percent higher in October 2020 than in October 2019, female deaths increased by 83 percent. One reason for this is that more women than men were working part-time in hotels, restaurants, and retail stores, where there were major layoffs. Another reason is that more women than men (27 percent compared with 10 percent) reported increased mental health challenges during the pandemic, according to the international aid organization CARE.[35]

Train Crossings

When people think of jump sites, they picture bridges, tall buildings, and cliffs, but another type of jump site is train crossings. At train crossings it's not the distance of the fall but the speed of the train that proves deadly. Trains—whether freight trains passing through town or subway trains in a crowded city—are too big and have too much momentum for anyone to be able to stop them quickly.

Where I live, in Northern California, the suicide deaths of Silicon Valley high school students jumping in front of trains have been big news. There have been clusters of them, many concentrated in the Palo Alto area, near Stanford University. The tracks run close enough to Palo Alto High School and Gunn High School—both considered elite schools—that the trains can be heard from most classrooms. Moreover, they pass through frequently, every twenty minutes or so. One student told a reporter with the *Atlantic* that on the day that another Palo Alto High School student threw himself in front of a train, the warning whistle of subsequent trains was like the cannon that went off in *The Hunger Games* whenever somebody died. It had the same ominous effect.[36]

Some people have speculated that part of the problem is that high-achieving parents often are not home when their children need them. They can afford to take their children on expensive vacations, but they aren't readily available to provide daily support. The other part of the problem is the pressure that parents and others place on their children to excel. It isn't enough to get into college; it has to be a top-level college that enhances a young person's career prospects.

Before smart phones and social media existed, it took time for word to reach most people about a death. That is no longer true, however. Within minutes of a suicide, particularly the suicide of a young person, the news goes viral. Through Twitter, Facebook, Instagram, and other platforms, people hear about it and start checking their phones for updates. They learn details that they shouldn't, details that further the potential for copycat suicides.

Obviously, train crossings present a different set of challenges when it comes to preventing suicides than do bridges, tall buildings, and cliffs. Even so, solutions are possible. One is referred to as "grade separation," whereby the tracks in some areas are raised to eliminate dangerous street-level crossings. Another is to install so-called Z-gates, which require pedestrians to weave through chain-link fencing to access train tracks. A third solution, for subway trains, is clear, sliding doors that close whenever trains are out of the station and open only when a train arrives. All these solutions are expensive, which is why signage with a suicide prevention message and the Lifeline number are being tried first. As with signs on bridges, however, the effect is minimal. Among the more whimsical solutions is putting airbags on the front of locomotives. Instead of cowcatchers, which push cattle away and prevent a train from derailing, the bags deploy as soon as they come into contact with an object, such as a human body, cushioning the impact.

One strategy that has shown some promise is installing mood lighting in Japanese train stations. In 2009 the East Japan Railway Company began installing special blue lights above platforms in all twenty-nine stations on the Yamanote Line.[37] Blue is considered a calming color, associated with the sky and the sea. After the number of suicides on the railway's lines increased from forty-two in 2007 to sixty-eight in 2009, the lights were tried in an effort to sooth anyone who might be distressed. Hanging at the end of each platform, which typically is the most isolated and least trafficked area and the area where people are most likely to throw themselves in front of a speeding train, the lights are brighter than standard fluorescent bulbs and bathe the platforms in blue color. According to a 2013 study by researchers at the University of Tokyo, suicide attempts decreased by 84 percent over a ten-year period at stations where the lights were in place.[38] A follow-up study in 2014 found that nearby stations without the lights didn't experience an increase in suicides, meaning that suicidal people didn't go there instead.[39]

Adding to the argument in favor of the mood lighting is another 2013 study in which the authors found that suicides on Japanese railways increased after several days of bad weather. Hiroshi Kadotani, of Shiga University of Medical Science, and a team of researchers analyzed 971 suicides and suicide attempts from 2002 to 2006. They determined that a high proportion of them occurred after a series of cloudy and rainy days. "Light exposure (blue light or bright white light) in trains may be useful in reducing railway suicides, especially when consecutive days without sunshine are forecasted," the study concluded.[40]

Installing blue lights is relatively cheap—East Japan Railway spent $165,000 for the special lights on the Yamanote Line[41]—and several train stations in England have followed suit. Japan's commitment to reducing suicides in the country doesn't end there, however. Gates and chest-high suicide barriers are in place at many stations in Japan, and plans are moving forward to install them in every Tokyo station by 2032. The projected cost is high—$4.7 billion—largely because Tokyo has 243 train stations and the barriers are expensive but also because some stations lack the platform space or structural strength for them.[42] As a result, modifications have to be made. Suicides at the stations also have a significant financial cost, however, as they delay trains and disrupt the schedules of tens of thousands of commuters and other travelers.

Suicide-prevention advocates are following developments in Japan with interest. If the country is successful in preventing train suicides, it could serve as a model for the rest of the world.

CHAPTER 9

Success Story

A NUMBER OF THINGS HAVE CHANGED SINCE MY BOOK *The Final Leap: Suicide on the Golden Gate Bridge* was published in 2012. Chief among them is that at that time there weren't any concrete plans, much less funding, to install a physical suicide deterrent on the world's top suicide site. In 2008 the board of directors of the Golden Gate Bridge, Highway, and Transportation District approved the addition of a net on the world-famous span—the first time in history that board members took such action—but they didn't approve any money to pay for it. That was still the case four years later, when *The Final Leap* came out. The net remained a vision for everyone who had lost a loved one to the bridge, as well as for many others, myself included, who had advocated for a physical suicide barrier, but it was a long way from becoming a reality.

Flash forward to today. Work is close to completion on a marine-grade, stainless steel net under the bridge to prevent suicides. It extends twenty feet out on both sides of the 1.7-mile span, is twenty feet below the roadway, and totals 380,000 square feet—the size of seven football fields. *Net* is something of a misnomer, however. It is fairly rigid so that anyone who falls into it most likely will suffer broken bones, it has a special weave to trap arms and feet, and it is angled in such a way as to make climbing out of it difficult.

The decision to install a net rather than a taller railing as a suicide deterrent was made because the net wouldn't detract from views on the bridge, and it wouldn't be noticeable from afar because it would be unpainted and thus blend in with the surrounding fog. At that time, the thinking was that if anyone ended up in the net, a special Bridge District vehicle with a cherry-picker arm would be used to retrieve them. Since then, a better plan has been developed. Firefighters who are stationed in nearby Sausalito already are trained in cliff rescues, and the Bridge District paid for a special $824,000 training facility where first responders there could practice retrieving someone from the net using a mini crane, called a "davit," and harness. At best, their services won't be needed because the presence of the net will be sufficient to deter anyone from jumping. At worst, firefighters are ready to rescue someone if the need arises.

So how did we get here? What events transpired over the past ten years to make the net possible? There were many, all of them essential to the story.

First, despite signage, emergency phones, and additional surveillance equipment, suicides from the bridge not only continued but increased, as did suicide attempts. In 2013, 48 people jumped to their death from the bridge—an all-time high—including 10 people in the month of August. Another 118 people were stopped from jumping by Bridge Patrol and California Highway Patrol officers.[1]

One of the August deaths was that of 17-year-old Gabri Aparacio in Marin County. "If it wasn't for the easy access to the bridge, I believe my daughter would be alive today," her father told reporters. "It is too late for Gabri, but this net will save lives, and it will save the eternal grief that families like us have to live through."[2]

A month later, 18-year-old Kyle Gamboa jumped from the bridge. He logged onto his computer, learned that the bridge didn't have a suicide barrier, skipped school, drove an hour and a half from his home to the bridge, stopped his truck midspan, and leaped over the railing. "He just woke that morning, googled the Golden Gate Bridge, looked on YouTube, saw that he could jump off, drove out here, and did it," his mother, Kimberlyrenee Gamboa, told the board of the Bridge District. "He didn't show any signs to anyone that he intended to end his life, not even his closest friends."[3] Her final words echoed those of Gabri Aparacio's parents. "If a suicide barrier had been in place, our son would still be with us today."[4]

Following Kyle's death, his father, Manuel, made a point of attending each month's meeting of the Bridge District board, even though, because of the distance, he had to take a full day off work to do it. He sat in the first row of spectator seats, often with Kimberlyrenee at his side, and held a photo of Kyle on his lap. Other parents had testified before the board, but not with the same persistence.

In 2014 the number of deaths was down, to 39, but the number of thwarted attempts was up, to 161. Manuel and Kimberlyrenee Gamboa responded by launching a petition on Change.org asking people to support a suicide barrier on the Golden Gate Bridge. Within a few weeks, more than 150,000 people had signed it. This marked a significant shift from earlier days when opponents to a barrier outnumbered supporters.

Also in 2014, the Bridge District board voted to spend $30 million to install a permanent median on the bridge to separate northbound and southbound vehicle traffic. Fewer than forty people had been killed in head-on collisions on the bridge since its opening seventy-seven years earlier, but this was a major concern of motorists. The decision was followed by newspaper editorials that said it was time now for the board to address the far more deadly issue of bridge suicides, whose number was fifty times the number killed in head-on collisions.

One of the deaths in 2014 was that of the 27-year-old grandson of Bridge District board member and past president John Moylan. Up to that point, it had been possible for some board members to ignore the issue of bridge suicides, but after that it became intensely personal, not only for Moylan, who already supported a suicide barrier on the bridge, but also for his colleagues. Moylan died in 2021 at age 92, having lived to see the barrier started.

In 2015 there were 33 confirmed suicides from the bridge and 153 successful interventions. Bridge District staff and community members, most notably supporters of the Bridge Rail Foundation, an all-volunteer nonprofit organization whose board I have served on since 2013, began strategizing ways to pay for the net. Three primary sources were pursued: the local branch of the federal Metropolitan Transportation Commission (MTC), the State of California's Department of Transportation (Caltrans), and California's Mental Health Services Act (MHSA). The MTC agreed to provide $27 million, Caltrans put up $22 million, the Bridge District contributed $20 million, and the MHSA granted $7 million, for a total of $76 million, which was the estimated cost of the net.

In 2016 there were 39 confirmed suicides from the bridge and 184 people were stopped from jumping. After comprehensive design drawings were developed, the Bridge District issued a bid package for the work. Bidders were required to have experience with bridge construction, and it was noted that the Bridge District intended to keep one side of the bridge—either the east side, used by bicyclists, or the west side, used by pedestrians—open during construction. Also, the "maintenance travelers," movable platforms under the bridge used by painters and ironworkers, would have to be reconfigured to allow for the net.

Representatives from numerous companies attended the bidders' conference, but only two companies actually bid on the project. The rest said that the cost would far exceed $76 million, and even one of the two companies that did bid submitted a bid that was double that. Seeing no alternative, the Bridge District accepted the low bid, which was submitted by a partnership of Shimmick Construction in Oakland and Danny Construction in San Francisco.

In January 2017, contracts were signed and work began. The timeline for completion was four years, meaning that the net would be in place by January 2021. Ironically, four years was the length of time it had taken to build the whole bridge, but things had changed since 1937, when the bridge opened. More state and federal agencies were part of the permitting process now.

The four-year timeline didn't last long, however. Shortly after Shimmick started work, the company was sold to AECOM, a global design company in Los Angeles, which immediately wanted to renegotiate the terms of the original contract. Bridge District officials had little leverage since materials had been ordered, construction was under way, and subcontractors were working on the project. It took some convincing, but the MTC and Caltrans were committed to the net, as was the Bridge District board by this time, and the three entities agreed to split the additional cost. A new completion date—July 2023—and new project budget—$211 million—were approved.

Not surprisingly, the number of suicides and attempted suicides from the bridge continued uninterrupted. In 2017 there were 33 confirmed suicides and a record 245 interventions. The latter number was owing in part to the Bridge District's hiring of additional officers to patrol the span. In 2018 there were 31 suicides and 187 interventions, and in 2019 there were 30 suicides and 167 interventions.

One of the suicide victims in 2019 was the 26-year-old son of Robert Rosenthal. In 2005 Rosenthal, a reporter with the *San Francisco Chronicle*, had spearheaded the paper's seven-day, front-page, top-of-the fold series on Golden Gate Bridge suicides. That series, titled "Lethal Beauty," focused renewed attention on the problem and as much as anything was responsible for the Bridge District's decision in 2008 to erect a net on the bridge.

In 2020 two notable events occurred. First, Shimmick Construction was sold again, this time to Oroco Capital in Bethesda,

Maryland. The completion date was pushed back six months, and $6 million was added to the cost. The second event was the coronavirus. A public health order was issued in California that allowed work on the net to continue, while all public works projects that weren't deemed essential were stopped. Even so, some of the subcontractors in other states, including the actual fabricator of the net, closed temporarily for Covid-related reasons. Also, the Bridge District lost millions of dollars as revenues from bridge tolls dropped significantly because of reduced vehicle traffic, and ridership on district-run buses and ferries decreased as well.

What didn't stop were the deaths. Even with reduced bus service to the bridge and reduced auto, bicycle, and pedestrian traffic, people managed to get to the Golden Gate Bridge during the height of the pandemic and end their lives, or try to. In 2020 there were 28 suicides and 185 interventions. In 2021 there were 25 suicides and 198 interventions. In 2022 there were 22 confirmed suicides and 160 interventions.

The Grim Reality

Obviously, suicides aren't confined to bridges, much less to one bridge. Suicide rates are up across the United States, and jumps of all types account for only 5 percent of the total. Still, for some people jumping is the preferred means of suicide, even though it's not always quick or painless.

"Some people seem to think that jumping off the bridge is a light, airy way to end your life," says retired Marin County coroner Ken Holmes, who was the focus of my book *The Education of a Coroner*. "I'd like to dispel that myth. When you jump off the bridge, you hit the water hard. It's not a pretty death."[5]

Holmes knows that better than anyone. Until 1990 the bodies of Golden Gate Bridge jumpers were delivered to the coroner's office in San Francisco. Then Coast Guard Station Golden Gate moved to

Marin County, and bodies began to be delivered to the coroner's office there. That was when Holmes learned about the magnitude of the problem. Until then he had had no idea, in part because it had been the practice in San Francisco to lump all jumping deaths—from tall buildings, cliffs, bridges, and freeway overpasses—in one category rather than separate them.

It takes four seconds for a body traveling at a speed of 75 miles per hour to hit the cold, dark water of San Francisco Bay after falling from the Golden Gate Bridge. Upon impact, the outer body stops, while internal organs keep moving, tearing loose from their connections. The result is similar to that of a pedestrian who is struck by a car going that fast. Most people die on impact, but not everyone. Five percent of Golden Gate Bridge jumpers survive the fall, plunge deep into the water, and end up drowning, their last minutes filled with agony and terror.[6]

For those who argue that people who want to kill themselves should be allowed to do so, it's important to remember that when someone dies by suicide, it's not just the victims and their families who suffer. The impact on loved ones is the greatest, and their lives will never be the same, but they are far from the only people who are affected. There is also the impact of suicides on witnesses. Seeing someone jump is traumatic. One time a man leaped in front of a group of visiting Girl Scouts. Group leaders scrambled to find counseling services for the girls, many of whom were still shaking hours later.[7]

Then there is the effect of suicides on first responders. They are thought to be inured to death, or at least used to it, but some deaths exert a toll. US Coast Guard Station Golden Gate is one of the busiest Coast Guard stations in the country. Based in Marin County, it's responsible for retrieving the bodies of Golden Gate Bridge jumpers and delivering them to the coroner's office, an emotionally draining and thankless task that causes some crew members to resign. A Coast Guard commander told me that no one joins the Coast

Guard so that they can recover the bodies of bridge jumpers. They join in order to save lives.

The same is true for Bridge Patrol officers, who until relatively recently received little or no training in suicide prevention but were expected to talk down a potential bridge jumpers. (Today they receive forty hours of suicide-prevention training.) If they are successful, the elation only lasts until the next intervention, which sometimes is the same day. If they fail, the memory can stay with them forever.

"If you make contact and the person jumps, it's definitely harder," said Lisa Locati when I interviewed her for *The Final Leap*. Now retired, she was captain of the Bridge District's patrol force at the time. "I was there when two people jumped at the same time. That will always be with me."[8] That was in 1998, when two women, aged 22 and 51, from different cities and unknown to each other, ended up at the same spot on the bridge at the same moment, each planning to end her life. They talked with each other and then briefly with patrol officers before leaping to their death.

Kevin Briggs is a retired California Highway Patrol officer who patrolled the Golden Gate Bridge for years. By his count, he talked to at least two hundred people who were "over the rail," meaning that they had climbed over the four-foot-tall railing and were perched on the chord, a 32-inch-wide beam that is the last place to stand before jumping. He persuaded all but two not to jump, but those two still haunt him. "One guy actually turned and shook my hand three times," Briggs says. "The third time, he said, 'Kevin, sorry, I have to go,' and jumped. It wears on you for the rest of your days. I think a little piece of me went down with him."[9]

Lastly, there is the effect of suicides on society as a whole. Whether the person jumps, shoots themself, overdoses, or dies another way, all of us miss out on the skills and talents he or she had or could have developed—as a physician, firefighter, educator, artist, caregiver, or any of a number of other vocations. According to a report that Holmes and Bridge Rail Foundation issued jointly, covering a fifteen-year period, the most common occupation of Golden Gate Bridge jumpers was student. The second most common was teacher.[10]

One Case Remembered

On January 29, 1993, a 35-year-old father in Fremont, California, killed his wife, grabbed their 3-year-old daughter, and drove to the bridge. Bridge officials spotted him walking in a suspicious fashion close to the railing and carrying a bundle that they realized too late was a child. Before they could reach him, he threw little Kellie Paige over the side and then jumped himself.

Jerry Check was one of the Coast Guard crew members on duty at Station Golden Gate that day. In his six years of service he had responded to more than a few suicide jumps. "Of the over 30 bodies I recovered," he says, "this one was the worst. I did all I could to save her life—rescue breathing, CPR—but ultimately she died later that day." Today, 60 years old and living in Michigan, where he teaches middle school and works with special ed students, Check says, "I keep recalling the jumpers in my head." He also keeps in touch with many of his fellow crew members even though they are spread across the country. "They, too, have some trouble dealing with the memories," he says.[11]

Pam Carter was a nurse at Marin General Hospital when Kellie Paige's body was brought into the emergency room. The toddler was still alive, but barely, and doctors worked frantically to try and save her. Kellie's injuries were too great, however. Afterward, Carter took Kellie's body to the hospital's morgue. The thought of leaving the child on a cold slab was abhorrent, so Carter borrowed a crib and laid Kellie in it. Her words echo Check's. "That had to be the worst. This little thing, taken like that by her father, the person she loved and looked up to. It was awful."[12]

Kellie's father died shortly after hitting the water. Ken Holmes, in his capacity as coroner of Marin County, observed him lying on a stokes litter, covered by a blanket. When Holmes examined Kellie's dead body, she was still in the emergency room with an immobilization collar around her neck, an endotracheal tube in her mouth, a catheter below, and IV lines in one wrist and one ankle. Holmes investigated thousands of deaths in a career that spanned four decades, and he has never forgotten this one. "It was a horrible case for everyone involved," he says.[13]

Kellie Paige wasn't the only child who died after being thrown off the Golden Gate Bridge by a suicidal father. Earlier, a man had jumped after tossing his 4-year-old son over the railing, and several months after Kellie's death another man did the same with his 2-year-old boy. All three cases were overlooked in the debate regarding whether a physical suicide deterrent should be added to the iconic span. Opponents talked about freedom of choice—"If someone wants to jump, let them; it's their life"—but no one talked about three young victims who had no choice. They were murdered, and the Golden Gate Bridge was the weapon.

Looking Back—and Ahead

For many years, the most popular method of killing oneself in England was to stick one's head in the oven and turn on the gas. Then, in the 1960s, oil and natural gas deposits were discovered in the North Sea, and the majority of English homes converted from coal, which has a high carbon monoxide content, to natural gas, which is cheaper and much less toxic. With the conversion, the country's suicide rate decreased by 30 percent, and it has stayed there.[14] When it no longer was possible to die by breathing oven fumes, people didn't resort to another means.

Perhaps the most compelling argument for the effectiveness of a suicide deterrent, particularly in relation to the Golden Gate Bridge, was provided by a study conducted by Richard Seiden, an emeritus professor at UC Berkeley. He and a team of graduate students tracked what happened to 515 people who were stopped from jumping off the Golden Gate Bridge. Cross-checking a list provided by the California Highway Patrol with death-certificate records, Seiden found that 94 percent of thwarted bridge jumpers were still alive twenty-five years later or had died by means other than suicide. Fewer than 6 percent ended up killing themselves.[15] (In a follow-up study, Seiden found that half the people who drove cars to the Golden Gate Bridge and then jumped had crossed the Bay Bridge to get there. No one went the other way, crossing the Golden Gate Bridge in order to jump from the Bay Bridge, even though the latter at its apex is the same height.)[16]

According to Denis Mulligan, general manager of the Golden Gate Bridge District, a key factor in the decision to install a net rather than a taller railing was that there had been only one instance in which a person jumped into a net after it was installed. That was on a bridge in Ithaca, New York. Everywhere else, a net ended the problem.

Ironically, at one time the Golden Gate Bridge did have a net. During the bridge's construction Joseph Strauss, the chief engineer, ordered a net to be strung the entire length of the span to protect workers. It cost $120,000—the equivalent of $2 million in today's currency—and at various times nineteen workers fell into it and were saved (they became known, in the language of the day, as the Halfway-to-Hell Club). Ten others weren't so lucky. They were standing on a section of scaffolding when it broke loose from its moorings and tore through the net, sending the workers to their deaths. This occurred only four months before the bridge was completed, but Strauss didn't hesitate to spend another $120,000 to have a new net installed. Once the bridge opened in May 1937, the net was removed.

Only a few communities with suicide bridges have erected nets to stop people from jumping. Most have opted for a taller railing, and officials with the Golden Gate Bridge District considered increasing the height of the current, four-foot-high railing to eight feet to prevent suicides. In the end, however, they chose the net so that views from the bridge wouldn't be affected. The decision mirrored a decision that was made during the bridge's construction. The original plans called for a taller railing specifically to prevent suicides. At the last minute, however, it was decided to lower the railing in order to enhance the view. Some people believe that Strauss was responsible because he was only five feet tall and wanted to see over the side. More likely, though, it was Irving Morrow, an Oakland architect who consulted on the final design.

What neither Strauss nor Morrow knew was that suicide sites beckon suicidal people to them like a siren's call. Whether the site is a bridge, a cliff, a train crossing, or something else, an aura develops that exerts a magnetic pull. Since it opened, no site has developed a more fatal lure or a stronger pull than the Golden Gate Bridge. The setting is magnificent, and the view—of San Francisco, the bay, Angel Island, Alcatraz, and, in the distance, Berkeley, Oakland, and the East Bay hills—is breathtaking.

If you have ever walked across the Golden Gate Bridge, three things probably surprised you. The first is how much the bridge moves. At the time it was built, it was the longest single-suspension bridge in the world. Single-suspension brides sway like a clothes line, and the longer the bridge is, the more it sways. The second surprise is how far down it is to the water. The drop from the roadbed is 220 feet, equivalent to twenty-five stories. The Golden Gate Bridge was the first bridge in the world to be built at the mouth of a major harbor, so it had to be tall enough to allow large ships to pass underneath. The third surprise is how low the railing is. At only four feet, it can be surmounted by almost anyone, from a 5-year-old girl who climbed over it and jumped because her father told her to (he then jumped as well)[17] to people who are overweight and in their eighties.

Ann McGuire is one of fewer than forty people who are known to have survived a jump from the bridge. She said afterward, "They make it so easy. It's creepy, and it's sad, and it's unnecessary."[18]

Tomorrow and Ever After

As I write this, installation of the net on the Golden Gate Bridge is almost complete. Its final weight is 225,000 pounds, which might sound like a lot; however, that is insignificant relative to the weight of the bridge—the weight of the materials the bridge is made of plus the weight of the load it carries. For comparison, each of the two cables that connect the twin towers on the bridge weighs 22 million pounds.

By the time you read this, if not before, the dark history of the Golden Gate Bridge will be over. Families and friends probably won't know that their loved one who is troubled remains alive today because the world's top suicide site no longer exerts a deadly pull. They won't know, except in a general way, of the losses that many others have suffered, largely in anonymity. No thought will be given to the fact that the bridge is now safe from suicide, much less to the people whose ultimate sacrifice made this possible. That is the way things like this often are. At least, everyone will be able to enjoy a magnificent structure because the tragedies associated with it have ended.

CHAPTER 10

Ending Suicide

IN 2011 THE RADIO PROGRAM *Freakonomics* broadcast a segment called "The Suicide Paradox." It began by talking about a small tribe of indigenous people in the Amazon Rainforest called the Piraha. They live in huts, sleep on the ground, and hunt with bows and arrows.

A linguist named Dan Everett, from Bentley University in Waltham, Massachusetts, had been studying the Piraha for thirty years by that time. His own stepmother had died by suicide, and when he mentioned it to the Piraha, their reaction was unexpected, at least to Everett: they laughed.

"That's really funny to us," they said. "You mean, you people, you white people, shoot yourselves in the head? We kill animals; we don't kill ourselves." According to Everett, the Piraha find the concept of suicide inexplicable. Not that suicide is unknown among other Amazonian tribes; it's just unknown to the Piraha.

Everett told *Freakonomics,* "Some people have suggested that, well, it's because they don't have the stresses of modern life, but that's just not true. There is almost 100 percent endemic malaria among the people. They're sick a lot. . . . Seventy-five percent of the children die before they reach the age of five or six. These are astounding pressures."[1] Yet there are zero suicides among the Piraha. They are among the poorest people in the world with astronomical rates of infant mortality and malaria, but the thought of killing themselves never enters their minds.

The belief that suicide is directly related to the quality of life is a popular one. If that is true, though, Steve Leavitt of *Freakonomics* asks, why don't more people die by suicide? "If you think about it," he says, "the poorest people in the world, surviving on less than a dollar a day, having to walk three miles to get water and carry 70-pound packs of water back just to survive, and those people do everything they can to stay alive."[2]

In 2018 the *Economist* noted that the global suicide rate had dropped by 29 percent since 2000, while the suicide rate in the United States had increased by 18 percent. The reason for the disparity, according to the magazine, was that the quality of life had improved elsewhere but declined in the United States, especially for middle-aged white men without a college degree.[3]

On the face of it, that makes sense, especially since middle-aged white men in the United States have a higher suicide rate than most other groups. It's not the complete answer, however. For one thing, the majority of people in the United States don't fall into that category; they are younger, nonwhite, or female. To attribute the increase primarily to a group that is in the minority is questionable, the more so because suicide rates are up for virtually every group. It also misses the point.

If you live in a country where most people have access to food, housing, health care, educational opportunities, and employment but you are poor, uneducated, unemployed, homeless, or an oppressed minority or can't afford medical or dental treatment, your misery deepens. Everyone else is doing well, or so it seems—getting good jobs, buying new clothes, driving expensive cars, dining at fancy restaurants—while you are struggling to meet basic needs.

This is different than, say, the example of the Piraha, where every-one is in the same situation. External problems such as a civil war or a recession affect almost everyone, maybe not equally but to vary-ing degrees. In the absence of these, however, society has a way of attributing an individual's misfortune to a personal defect of some kind—a character flaw, physical disability, or mental health prob-lem—which adds to the person's depression. At a time when you are witnessing or hearing or reading about other people's successes—particularly in this age of social media, when few people post the bad things they are going through[4]—you are failing.

Henry Ford Behavioral Health

In my book *The Last and Greatest Battle: Finding the Will, Com-mitment, and Strategy to End Military Suicides*, I say that I believe it's possible to end suicides among active-duty service members and veterans if the military adopts many of the principles of Henry Ford Behavioral Health, a division of Henry Ford Health in Detroit. I ac-knowledge that the solution isn't simple. On the contrary, it re-quires institutional changes in policies, procedures, attitudes, and cultures at two of our biggest bureaucracies, the Departments of Defense and Veterans Affairs. It also isn't cheap. Nevertheless, it's possible.

In 2001 Henry Ford Behavioral Health implemented a new, un-tested, systemwide approach to suicide. The aim was to eliminate patient suicides. Not reduce the number of patients who kill them-selves, but eliminate suicides altogether.

Henry Ford Health is a health maintenance organization, which means that its patients are covered by private health care insurance. At the time, the behavioral health division comprised two hospitals, nine clinics, and five hundred employees. One would expect a lower rate of suicide among its patients than among the general population, many of whom lack private coverage. In fact, though, until 2001 the suicide rate at Henry Ford was 89 per 100,000 patients, more than seven times the national average.

The suicide rate at Henry Ford can be explained partly by the fact that the focus of behavioral health care systems is treating people who are mentally ill, so their patient population is more at risk for suicide than the population in general. Even so, an abnormally high percentage of patients at Henry Ford were killing themselves, which was enough to alarm Dr. C. Edward Coffey, CEO of Behavioral Health. Coffey rounded up every employee in the system to brainstorm ways to reduce the number of suicides. Initial conversations focused on what constituted success. Was it reducing the suicide rate within the system by half, or to the level of the national rate, or even lower?

According to Coffey, if 99.9 percent accuracy is good enough, then twelve babies in the United States will be given to the wrong parents every day, more than eighteen thousand pieces of mail will be mishandled every hour, and two million records will be lost every year by the Internal Revenue Service.[5] One Henry Ford employee said that even a single suicide was unacceptable if it was your child, and that helped set the target—zero. In other words, the goal was perfection, not a single suicide among Henry Ford's thousands of patients.

In sports, perfection is achieved sometimes. There are perfect games in baseball, when no batter reaches base, and perfect games in bowling, when someone throws twelve consecutive strikes. A basketball player may make all of his or her shots in a game, and a golfer may shoot a hole in one. In the realm of health care, however, perfection is rare, and it's even rarer to establish it as a goal. Aside from its being thought to be unattainable, there is a fear that setting the bar so high will lead to disappointment when people fail to reach it, regardless of how much progress they make along the way. It's better, the thinking goes, to set goals that are a stretch but have a reasonable chance of being met. This way everyone feels good about the outcome.

That thinking didn't deter Dr. Coffey and his team. They decided to aim for perfection anyway, and in so doing they learned something surprising and valuable. Rather than being discouraged by a goal that seemed unreachable, employees were energized by it. They committed to it in a way that has affected the whole system since then. "Pursuing perfection is no longer a project or initiative for our team," Coffey said later, "but a principal driving force embedded in the fabric of our clinical care."[6]

After setting the goal, Behavioral Health began developing a plan to achieve it. The first step was to establish a consumer advisory panel to work with staff in designing the program. Since the program was aimed at patients, it seemed only natural and appropriate to get patient input. Next was the program itself. It was decided that every patient admitted to a Behavioral Health facility would be assessed for risk of suicide. Specific interventions were then crafted for three different levels of risk. Every employee who had patient contact was required to take a course in suicide prevention and score 100 percent on a written test—perfection—or retake it.

The real work followed. Institutional changes were made so that patients had access to immediate help and information through email communications with doctors, drop-in prescription pickups, and same-day medical appointments. In addition, protocols were devised and implemented to temporarily remove firearms from a patient's home if the person was determined to be a suicide risk.

The results were dramatic. In four years patient suicides at Henry Ford dropped by 75 percent, to 22 per 100,000 people.[7] It would have been easy to stop there, but Henry Ford didn't. By 2009 the system had gone two and a half years without a single suicide among its patient population. The commitment to perfection from the top down and the bottom up made the difference.[8]

Ending suicides in a large behavioral health care system is impressive, but it's not the same as ending them throughout the country. It's important to note, though, that the source of Henry Ford's success wasn't the singular vision of its leader, the quality of its patient care prior to the "zero suicide" program being implemented, or the zeal and dedication of its staff. Certainly Dr. Coffey was visionary, the program was well designed, and many employees worked hard at it. Those weren't the key, however. The key was everyone's commitment to the goal. The staff at Henry Ford not only accepted the challenge, they embraced it. They believed that striving for perfection was important and were determined to achieve it.

The Zero Suicide Model

The success of Henry Ford's efforts inspired other health care providers to follow suit. In 2012 a partnership formed between the US Office of the Surgeon General and the National Action Alliance for Suicide Prevention. The latter is made up of 250 organizations that are committed to advancing the National Strategy for Suicide Prevention, which focuses on best practices in the areas of screening, safety planning, and support. At the center of the strategy is Zero Suicide, a framework that embodies lessons learned from Henry Ford. There are seven specific elements, of which leading system-wide cultural change is the first. Leadership starts at the top, and key executives must be early champions, able to persuade staff that it's possible to end suicides while also fostering a blame-free environment so that that can happen.

The second element is training a competent and caring workforce. Interactions with staff are a critical part of any patient's experiences with a health care provider, and this is even more true for suicidal patients. Their previous experiences may have been less than satisfactory or even nonexistent. It's imperative that staff be confident in their abilities as well as compassionate in their approach, and this is the result of training. According to the Zero Suicide website, "Any door must be the right door through which the staff, both clinical and non-clinical, engage people at risk by encouraging them to believe treatment can work, that the staff care about them, and instilling a commitment to come back to the next appointment."[9]

Third is identifying individuals at risk of suicide. This means assessing patients for risk of suicide as part of every visit to a health care provider. Regardless of the reason for the visit—illness, aches, a broken bone—they are screened to determine whether there is any suicidal ideation or planning. People doing the screening not only need a good assessment tool; they need to be able to ask about suicide without conveying discomfort or judgment.

Fourth is engaging suicidal patients in safety planning. Patients not only work with counselors to develop safety plans specific to the patient's needs—plans that take into account the most timely, appropriate, and culturally relevant treatment options available for that individual—but commit to following through.

Fifth is treating people at risk of suicide. This can consist of a single in-person session, but more likely it involves multiple sessions and perhaps different techniques. Because some suicidal people are ambivalent in their approach to life, it's up to the counselor to help them find a solution to their pain that doesn't include suicide. Whether it's cognitive behavioral therapy (CBT), in which accurate, positive thoughts replace negative and faulty thinking; dialectical behavior therapy (DBT), an offshoot of CBT pioneered by psychologist Masha Linehan that focuses on helping people accept the reality of their lives and behaviors in order to change them; or cognitive processing therapy (CPT), in which traumatic events are processed through written narratives and restructured assessment (a common form of therapy for military members suffering from PTSD), these or other evidence-based treatment programs are tools for treating suicide.

Sixth is transitioning suicidal individuals following psychiatric hospitalization to other providers who can provide longer-term support. As noted in chapter 1, people who have been hospitalized are most at risk in the week immediately following discharge, and seeing that they have follow-up care is essential. Providers can check in with them regularly, remind them of appointments, and provide support between appointments, if necessary, so that treatment continues.

The last element is improving policies and procedures in order to keep up with developments in the field and provide the most effective services possible. Collecting and examining data is a large part of this, but so too is creating an environment that offers support rather than criticism to clinicians when patients attempt or die by suicide. Learning from failures in care can be as important as celebrating successes.

The Zero Suicide model is a joint effort of the US Department of Health and Human Services, the Substance Abuse and Mental Health Services Administration, Universal Health Services, the Suicide Prevention Resource Center, the National Action Alliance for Suicide Prevention, and the Education Development Center. It's being adopted by a growing number of hospitals, mental health clinics, and other health care providers with favorable results.

According to a 2021 study led by the New York State Office of Mental Health, "Large-scale implementation of the Zero Suicide model is associated with lower suicidal behaviors of patients under care."[10] As reported in the *Psychiatric News*, researchers assessed practices at 110 mental health clinics in New York State and found that those most closely allied to the Zero Suicide model had the fewest suicide attempts and deaths. In particular, "having suicide care embedded in the medical chart, written clinical workflows for suicide care, and data collection and review by clinical teams," in combination with efforts to reduce patients' access to lethal means at home, had the biggest impact.[11]

A study published in the *British Journal of Psychiatry* in 2021 reached the same conclusion. On the basis of information pertaining to 604 people in Australia who had made one or more suicide attempts, researchers determined that those who had received multilevel care according to the Zero Suicide framework made fewer subsequent attempts than did others. This was true across all groups regardless of demographic differences.[12]

The Zero Suicide model is proving to be an effective way for health care providers to reduce and in many cases prevent future suicides; however, the responsibility to end suicides isn't limited to medical and mental health professionals. All segments of society have a role to play.

What Individuals Can Do

It is important for people to start talking openly and honestly about suicide, to stop hiding it and instead cast a light. For individuals, this means dusting off family skeletons and having frank conversations about the death of a relative or close friend. It means using appropriate terminology, words that are empathic and foster help-seeking rather than words that are judgmental and contribute to stigma. It also means helping others to understand the impact of suicide on our society.

Two traveling exhibits that include strong visual representations have raised public awareness of suicide. The exhibit "Send Silence Packing," a project of Active Minds, a nonprofit organization based in Washington, DC, comprises twelve hundred backpacks, photos, and other personal items donated by family members and friends of college students who died by suicide. One of the organizers explained, "A backpack is a very personal item. It's something that all students have, and it's something that all students can relate to."[13]

The traveling exhibit "Whose Shoes," organized by the Bridge Rail Foundation, in the San Francisco Bay Area, features the footwear of hundreds of people who have jumped off the Golden Gate Bridge. Hearing a number, whether it's one thousand, two thousand, or more, isn't nearly as effective as seeing a huge display of shoes spread out before you, representing a vast canvas of lives lost.

People who are motivated can be trained in suicide prevention. Many individuals have taken a class in CPR, but the odds of seeing someone have a heart attack or stroke are smaller than the odds of knowing someone who is contemplating suicide and preparing to act. This isn't to minimize the value of knowing first aid but rather to emphasize the importance of skill building in preventing suicides.

Better yet, people can volunteer for training in answering calls or responding to texts to their local suicide hotline. Volunteers are always needed, and there are many personal benefits. First, they are helping others. The opportunity to impact people's lives in such an important and positive way—especially people one doesn't know—is rare. Second, they learn valuable crisis-management skills that can help them in their everyday life. In interactions with family members, friends, colleagues, or clients, the importance of being able to listen, express empathy, and help troubleshoot someone's problems without judging them can't be overestimated. Third, answering calls on a suicide hotline helps put one's own problems in perspective. What might otherwise seem unmanageable can pale in comparison to the obstacles that many hotline callers face. Lastly, a camaraderie often develops among people who are attracted to this kind of work. Phone counselors become an extended family, caring for and supporting one another.

Another avenue is to learn whether there are any suicide hotspots in your community, such as a bridge, a tall building, a cliff, or a train crossing, and advocate for a physical barrier to prevent future jumps. Nearly every successful effort to erect a barrier at a jump site has started with a small group of people—or sometimes just one person—determined to end unnecessary deaths from that location.

Lobbying for suicide-prevention services and funding is always good. Send letters to the editors of publications that report on suicide, praising them for increasing awareness and following established media guidelines or pointing out their publication's failing and missed opportunity if they don't. Write or call local elected officials and tell them that suicide prevention is an important issue and merits their attention and support.

If nothing else, parents whose children play at other people's homes should get in the habit of asking whether there are any guns in the house. Gun owners, in turn, shouldn't feel offended by the question but should treat it as an opportunity to demonstrate responsible gun ownership by locking their weapons and storing ammunition separately.

In a few instances, a single individual has had a profound impact. In Australia, the highest suicide rate is in Tasmania, where a woman named Amanda Johnson lost three close friends and nine other acquaintances to suicide. To deal with her grief, she started asking friends to check in each day at 4:00 p.m. and report how they were feeling on a simple scale of 1 to 10. The reports were shared among the group and facilitated an active support network. The concept was such a success that Johnson turned it into a free phone app called Be a Looper, referring to keeping people "in the loop." The app quickly spread around the world and in 2018 was nominated for a Global Mobile Award.[14]

Another creative app inventor is Tyler Skluzacek. He was 13 when his father, a US Army veteran, returned from Iraq in 2006 clearly changed. "He used to be so active and happy," Tyler told *CNN*, but after the war he was "depressed, lethargic, irritable, and the worst part is he wasn't sleeping." Because of nightmares from his time in the service, Patrick Skluzacek said, "I was scared of closing my eyes." The only way he was able to sleep was to consume alcohol and swallow pills before going to bed. Drinking more and more, he lost his wife, then their home.

In 2015, when he was a senior in college, Tyler created a smartwatch app that tracks, manages, and stops nightmares. It uses a person's heart rate and movements to detect nightmares, then emits gentle vibrations to pull them out of it without waking them up. "In that moment, my entire life changed," Patrick said. "All of a sudden, everything stopped. I was sleeping so much better."[15]

In 2017 Tyler sold rights to the app, now called Nightware. At last report, it was available with a physician's prescription as a therapeutic device primarily to treat PTSD and came preinstalled on an Apple Watch.

What Clergy Can Do

Clergy have a different role. They can talk regularly about mental health issues as a way of combating stigma. They also can get training in dealing with these issues because even though they don't graduate from seminary as mental health counselors, often they are put in a position where this is expected of them. One former pastor, following the suicide of a church leader in California and remembering his own suicide attempt earlier in life, said, "Churches need to look more like psych wards." By this he meant that they need to adopt a realistic approach to meeting the mental health needs of their members. "'I'm praying for you' is not a solution," he said, "even though it feels like the right thing to say."

He recommends that pastors keep a list of local mental health counselors, post it with announcements, and save it on their smartphone for the next time someone comes to them in crisis. He also encourages churches to offer rent-free space to therapists in exchange for mental health training of church staff and reduced-fee therapy for members of the congregation.[16] Both are good suggestions and fairly simple to implement.

What Schools Can Do

When 22-year-old Katie Meyer killed herself in her dorm room at Stanford University in 2021, it sent shockwaves across the San Francisco Bay Area and the country. As the star goalkeeper for the women's soccer team Meyer had helped Stanford win the national championship two years earlier. Moreover, she was the fourth Stanford student to die by suicide in just over a year. Stanford officials vowed to improve mental health services at the school, in part by hiring four more counselors and therapists. Eighteen months after Meyer's death, however, all four positions remained unfilled, and the clinical staff were overwhelmed.[17]

Most colleges offer mental health counseling for students, but owing to staff shortages it tends to be underfunded, poorly promoted, and difficult to access. Assessing the need for mental health services, developing a comprehensive strategy for meeting the need, and establishing clear procedures for what to do if a student is in crisis or hospitalized enables school counselors, medical staff, and administrative leaders to act quickly and effectively to prevent suicides. At a minimum, the counseling center should be housed in an area with other student services so that it's visible and accessible and students don't feel awkward going there. Beyond that, the center can provide phone consultations, text and chat services, evening and drop-in appointments, and referrals to off-campus resources for long-term and crisis situations. If staffing is a problem, a college can consider using interns and peer counselors linked to the community and provide them with clinical supervision and training.

It's not just colleges that are experiencing a mental health crisis among students, however. High schools and junior highs are too, and they don't have anywhere near the financial resources of a top university like Stanford, with its multi-billion-dollar endowment. Fortunately, a significant part of the solution doesn't depend on finances as much as it depends on having a plan.

There are three stages in dealing with any crisis. The first is prevention, which involves taking steps to reduce the likelihood of a crisis occurring. The primary focus is risk assessment. In school settings this means evaluating each student's mental health, identifying those who now or in the near future may be contemplating suicide, and seeing that they receive appropriate treatment as soon as possible. It's an ongoing process that requires well-thought-out assessment tools, good training practices, and a competent and confident staff. It also requires that staff ask parents whether their child has access to firearms, medication, or other lethal means.

The second stage is intervention, which involves taking action to stop a crisis from escalating and providing first aid or other support to any victims. Intervention starts with getting the facts and assessing the situation, then sharing information among predetermined, need-to-know individuals. After that, everyone follows established policies for how school personnel respond to in-school and out-of-school suicide attempts, as well as when parents are notified, when law enforcement is summoned, and when students can return to school following an incident. Many schools have plans to deal with bullying, but fewer have plans to deal with suicide.

The third stage, postvention, begins when the immediate crisis is over. It includes initiating support services, such as grief counseling. It also includes communicating externally, primarily via the media, by a designated spokesperson, who provides basic facts free of judgment. This serves to control rumors and avoid sensationalized reporting. In addition, postvention includes appropriate memorials. All deaths should be treated with reverence but also with messaging that minimizes the possibility of suicide contagion. In this way postvention becomes prevention, and the cycle starts all over again.

What Businesses Can Do

There are multiple opportunities for businesses to contribute to the solution. Physicians can cut back on prescriptions for highly addictive painkillers and medications for which a side effect is increased risk of suicide. Pharmaceutical companies can package over-the-counter medications in modest amounts and in such a way that a large number of pills can't be dispensed at one time. Gun shops can post information about suicide, including the 988 Suicide and Crisis Lifeline's phone number, and ask anyone who is buying a gun for the first time what they plan to use it for, strongly suggest that they get training, and encourage them to store it safely.

One innovative approach is being led by a group of architects in New York City. They are advocating that the Uniform Building Code, which mandates standards for public safety in the design and construction of all permanent structures throughout most of the United States, be modified to include suicide prevention. Their effort was prompted by four suicides at a newly constructed tourist site in Manhattan's Hudson Yards called the Vessel. It opened to the public in 2019 and consists of a spiral staircase wound in a honeycomb-like structure that is 150 feet above the ground at the top. After three people jumped to their death from the structure in the first two years, it was closed to the public while various preventative measures were considered, including adding netting or glass barriers. These changes ultimately weren't made, however. Instead, there were minor modifications and the structure reopened in 2021 with the requirement that all visitors be accompanied by at least one person. Two months later a 14-year-old boy jumped to his death while he was there with his family, and the Vessel closed indefinitely.

The chairman of the community board that includes the area where the Vessel is located said, "Technically, it is a work of art, but we are dealing with life-and-death issues. Art and architecture have to take a back seat."[18] At the time of this writing, local officials are testing safety nets around the Vessel, but the structure remains closed. That just adds more credence to the idea that making changes to the Uniform Building Code to prevent future suicides has significant potential not only in cities like New York but in communities across the country.

Another way that businesses can help is to be visible, vocal advocates for suicide prevention. One example is Sip of Hope in Chicago, which bills itself as "the world's first coffee shop where 100 percent of the proceeds support proactive suicide prevention and mental health education." The message on its website is affirming and supportive: "Life is hard and some days we need more than a cup of coffee to get us through the day. We need to remind ourselves that despite the things we've been through, it's okay to feel pain, it's okay to talk about it. The biggest obstacle to preventing suicide is silence. We as a community can start the conversation about mental health; we are in this together. Prevention starts with a conversation, and the conversation starts here." In addition to coffee, Sip of Hope sells T-shirts in a variety of styles bearing the shop's catchphrase, "It's OK not to be OK."

A second example is Tiny Turnip, a philanthropically minded apparel company in southern California. In 2018 the brother-in-law and best friend of baseball superstar Mike Trout killed himself at age 24. Trout's wife, Jessica, struggled to talk about his death, not just publicly but with relatives and friends. Then she met Jalynne Crawford, the wife of San Francisco Giants shortstop Brandon Crawford, whose 38-year-old sister had died from an asthma attack. The two women bonded in their grief, with the Crawfords telling the Trouts about Tiny Turnip. In 2020 the Trouts partnered with the company to market a T-shirt that featured a baseball and glove styled as a semicolon with the message "Your game isn't over yet." A semicolon is a metaphor for suicide prevention in that it marks where a sentence could end but doesn't. Proceeds from sales of the shirts go to the American Foundation for Suicide Prevention.[19]

Another example is a farmer in Wisconsin who turned eleven acres of his cornfield into a billboard for suicide prevention. Carved into the field was a maze with the message "Your life matters" and the Lifeline number. "Everybody is somebody's most important person," said John Govin, who owns the field. "If we can make a difference, if we save a life this fall, that's worth it." Mazes are an annual tradition in the area, and Govin told reporters that he and his wife always pick a theme that has meaning to their family. In 2019 the theme was suicide because it was, in Govin's words, "something we, unfortunately, had to face."[20] People pay to walk through the mazes, and a percentage of the profits goes to suicide prevention.

On a larger scale, Hyatt Hotel heir John Pritzker and his former wife, Lisa Stone Pritzker, donated $60 million of the $235 million needed to construct a five-story, state-of-the-art mental health facility in San Francisco. Designed to bring multiple campuses and disciplines under one roof, it's closely affiliated with the University of California San Francisco Benioff Children's Hospital and the world-renowned Langley Porter Psychiatric Institute. Named the Nancy Friend Pritzker Psychiatry Building after John's sister, a Stanford graduate who took her life in 1972—when few people talked about mental illness, including members of her family—it's set up to serve patients from early childhood to early adulthood, including those with serious disorders who haven't responded to standard treatments.

At one time, Lisa Stone Pritzker volunteered on the psychiatric floor at San Francisco General Hospital, and she was shocked to see that the waiting room was dark and windowless and that traumatized children under age 5 were seated next to deeply disturbed adults. That has changed with the new building, which has separate entrances and separate departments for children and features natural light and cheerful décor. "This building was designed with stigma in mind," says John Pritzker. It's filled "with light and art and not like any other building in the behavioral sciences."[21]

What Public-Private Partnerships Can Do

One weekday night in 2018 a man threatened to jump from a freeway overpass in Detroit. Michigan State Police quickly closed down all twelve lanes of traffic in both directions on Interstate 696, then rerouted thirteen semitrucks to form a tight line under the overpass. That way, if the man jumped, he would fall only five or six feet onto the top of one of the trucks, rather than fifteen feet onto a passing car or the roadway. The man didn't jump. Instead he was talked down.[22] It was an example of a public entity—Michigan State Police—collaborating with a private entity—independent truckers—to save someone's life.

Another example of public-private collaboration is occurring in a few places across the country and needs to be replicated everywhere. Public and private agencies are sharing information they have collected on suicides and suicide attempts, suppressing identifying characteristics to preserve individuals' anonymity but making it possible to aggregate data for tracking, reporting, and public policy purposes.

In 2018 the National Institute of Mental Health funded the development of the Maryland Suicide Data Warehouse with the aim of linking various sources of data to analyze and prevent suicide deaths. At present the project, led by Johns Hopkins University, has data from 2012 to 2017 on roughly five million Maryland residents, including hospital and emergency discharges from five select health systems, medical examiner data, and health data related to housing, employment, education, income, and crime. Continuing to analyze and refresh the data, as is planned, will improve suicide risk identification and reduce the number of suicides, experts believe.

On a smaller scale is an innovative partnership formed in Santa Clara County, California, led by the county public health department. Four separate governmental entities—public health, mental health (which operates Santa Clara's suicide hotline), the hospital system, and the coroner's office—have begun sharing suicide data. Stanford University, which is in the county and has its own hospital and behavioral health care system, is part of the collaborative and provides data too. In addition, Stanford professors and graduate students are assisting county staff in analyzing the information that is collected.

One of the first reports issued in Santa Clara included a breakdown of suicides by city the previous year. It attracted widespread attention, especially in communities where suicide had not been believed to be a problem. One police chief took umbrage at the report, saying that it noted three suicides in his small city, when there hadn't been any. Researchers showed him the data, and the police chief was forced to admit that he was wrong.

It's worth noting that when Santa Clara launched the project, the county already had the lowest suicide rate (7.5 per 100,000 people) in California. That didn't stop county officials from doing more, though.[23]

What State Officials Can Do

In San Diego, $14 million has been approved for the design of a stainless steel net on the Coronado Bridge, the second-deadliest bridge in the United States after the Golden Gate. This approval came after the installation of four-inch-tall metal bird spikes on the bridge's railing had no effect in reducing suicides. The net—more like a horizontal mesh fence—will extend eight to ten feet above the existing concrete railing, attached to posts, and run the length of the bridge. It is estimated to cost $130 million, and construction is supposed to start in 2026 and be completed in 2029.[24]

In Washington, DC, the Department of Transportation announced in January 2023 that it was moving forward with plans to install a permanent suicide barrier on the Taft Bridge, which averages one suicide a year. Earlier efforts to end suicides from the bridge met resistance from several historic preservation groups; however, these groups no longer oppose a barrier. Funding has been allocated for the design, which could be a fence or a net, depending on the final decision, with construction starting as soon as 2024.

In Tennessee, temporary fencing was installed in 2022 on the Natchez Trace Parkway Bridge, sometimes referred to as the Double Arch Bridge, in Franklin. Completed in 1994, the bridge received the 1995 Presidential Award for Design Excellence, but it has been a site for suicide ever since. At present the National Park Service is considering plans for a permanent suicide barrier, but until its construction is under way the temporary fence will remain.

Meanwhile, a 2019 study by the New Mexico Department of Transportation concluded that building a higher railing on the Rio Grande Gorge Bridge, northwest of Taos, would save lives. The bridge is one of the tallest spans in the country—six hundred feet above the Rio Grande—and has been the site of at least fifty suicides since records started being kept in 1991. Like the Golden Gate Bridge, it's an engineering marvel, attracting visitors from around the world because of its breathtaking setting, and the railing is only four feet high.

"The bridge is a spectacular expression of human ingenuity," states an editorial in the *Santa Fe New Mexican*, a leading newspaper in the state. "It is a draw for tourists and moviemakers because of its visual impact. Yet it has become a place of sadness. Addressing that problem, more than beauty or historic significance, is what matters." To date, however, neither the governor nor the state legislature has expressed interest in pursuing a taller railing. Until they do, "more people will die," the editorial concludes.[25]

Maryland's Chesapeake Bay Bridge also was hailed as an engineering marvel when it opened in 1952. It was the longest continuous steel structure over water in the world at that time. Two months later, the first suicide occurred from the bridge. Bridge authorities didn't begin keeping track of bridge suicides until sixteen years later, but since then there have been at least eighty suicides and nearly the same number of nonfatal attempts. Over the years, surveillance cameras, emergency call boxes, and suicide-prevention signage have been added, with no effect. Meanwhile, calls for a physical barrier have been ignored by state officials.[26]

In Oregon, people want more done to prevent suicides from the Astoria-Megler Bridge, connecting Astoria, Oregon, to Point Ellice, near Megler, Washington, which currently has only signage and crisis phones. Among the options are changes to a deck-level gate, currently topped by barbed wire, that allows access to the top of the bridge. People have been able to bypass the gate to get to the span's highest point and jump. The addition of fencing or a net is one of several options under consideration, but as of this writing there has been no further progress.[27]

The story is similar in Newport County, Rhode Island. A 2021 bill titled "Bridging the Gaps for Safety" called for suicide barriers on three bridges there that collectively have been the site of more than two dozen deaths since 2010.[28] The Rhode Island Turnpike and Bridge Authority said that more study was needed to determine whether the bridges could withstand the weight of barriers, however. This is a common stalling tactic that was made more apparent when an $82.5 million federal grant in 2022 to make upgrades to state bridges for safety reasons did not include physical barriers. To date, more than six thousand people have signed an online petition calling for suicide barriers on four Rhode Island bridges. So far, their call for action has been unanswered, although advocates there remain optimistic that it will be one day.[29]

The list goes on. In Milwaukee, suicide prevention advocates are lobbying for a barrier on the Hoan Bridge after forty people jumped to their death between 2003 and October 2022. The New York State Bridge Authority, which is responsible for six bridges in Upstate New York, is looking into suicide barriers after several suicides in 2021 and 2022. Spokane, Washington, is considering a protective barrier on the Monroe Street Bridge following four suicides in nine days.[30]

The point is that the pattern tends to be the same in every community. Awareness is raised, people express concerns, the local transportation authority is pressured to do something, and if the outcry is loud enough, signage is posted, emergency phones are installed, and people are encouraged to call a local or national hotline number if they are feeling suicidal. These efforts, while well intentioned, are largely ineffective. Anything short of a physical barrier is futile in addressing the problem. Barriers might seem expensive, especially if they are added years after a bridge is built rather than incorporated into the original design, but to anyone who has lost a loved one because a jump site didn't have a tall railing or a net to prevent suicides, the cost is insignificant relative to the unending pain and suffering they endure.

Moreover, suicide barriers can be cost effective. In an April 2022 report published in *JAMA Network Open*, a journal of the American Medical Association, researchers in Australia determined that if barriers were installed on multiple bridges across their country, they would return the equivalent of $2.40 in US currency for every $1 invested, or $270 million over ten years. The savings would be "due to averted suicides over the intervention cost," meaning that the cost of responding to suicides and suicide attempts was more than double the cost of barriers. Economically, the installation of barriers on bridges "is a warranted strategy for suicide prevention," the report concluded.[31]

What Federal Officials Can Do

In 1975 Washington, DC, enacted a law that made it harder to obtain handguns. The result was a 23 percent drop in the rate of suicide by firearms. There were no associated increases in suicide by other means, and the effects were found only in Washington, DC, not in neighboring states.[32]

Universal background checks and ten-day waiting periods to buy a firearm can be mandated. The sale of high-caliber automatic weapons can be banned. States can enact so-called red flag laws, which authorize police and immediate family members to remove firearms from people deemed to be a threat to themselves or to others. In Indiana, researchers determined that this simple act reduced suicides by 7.5 percent.[33] In 2019 California passed a bill to strengthen the law by giving coworkers, teachers, and school staff the ability to ask a judge for this right as well. As of 2023, nineteen states and the District of Columbia had some sort of red flag law; however, the majority of states did not.

Physical barriers can be erected at bridges and other known jump sites. Federal legislation exists that mandates the installation of stop signs and stop lights at intersections where traffic is unregulated and fatal accidents have occurred. The same thinking can be applied to jump sites: after a certain threshold is reached, whether it's one or five or ten suicides at a site, then the local community could be required to erect a barrier of some kind. The barrier might be a tall railing or a net, but it must be physical. We don't expect a sign on a steep, mountain road to keep people from driving over the side. If drivers don't see it or don't take it seriously, if the road is wet or they are intoxicated, it won't help. That is why there are guardrails.

Legislation passed in 2012 specifically authorizes the use of federal money to install safety barriers on bridges and at railroad crossings.[34] In 2019 bipartisan legislation was introduced in Congress to fund a federal grant program for barriers and nets on bridges and to study other possible measures to reduce suicides by jumping. The legislation, called the Barriers to Suicide Act, had twenty-six co-sponsors but wasn't heard before the 116th Congress ended in 2021.[35]

Meanwhile, the National Park Service can require all rangers to receive training in suicide prevention. Prisons can commit to min-imizing the time that individual inmates spend in solitary confine-ment. Police associations can require law enforcement officers to receive suicide-prevention training and make sure that counseling is provided anytime there is a suicide by cop, even if the officers in-volved don't think they need it.

In 2019, after New York City experienced it's seventh suicide by a police officer in the first six months of the year, the mayor, a po-lice commissioner, and other city officials pleaded with officers who were struggling with suicidal thoughts to come forward and talk about them. "You may not know this," they told the officers, "and it may be hard to imagine, but you are not out there all by yourself."[36] By October, there had been three more NYPD suicides, making ten for the year to that point, which was double the annual average of four or five. The 2019 suicide rate of police officers in New York also was double that of civilians in the city.[37]

It's not enough just to say that it's okay to seek help. Between the sixth and tenth suicides, New York City's Department of Investiga-tions reported, internal support services in the police department were "underused" because the stigma of asking for help was too strong. "It's probably part of the cop thing, keeping in your emotions" said a longtime homicide detective in San Diego who compiled a book of real-life notes left by suicidal people.[38]

The report recommended mandatory mental health checks for all officers,[39] which is a start, but only that. The real answer is to implement widespread, institutional changes that break down stigma and make self-care an important and accepted part of com-munity policing.

What the Military Can Do

There are many things that the Departments of Defense and Veterans Affairs can do to end suicides by active-duty service members and vets. One relatively simple step is to ban the practice of allowing troops to take their weapons home with them when they are off duty, as was done in Israel. Another is to allow health care professionals to ask troops and reservists living off-base if they have a firearm at home. Beyond that, broad changes in attitudes and culture are needed within both departments.

When combat veterans come home, they bring the war with them. They make constant perimeter checks to ensure the safety of family members. They limit outside activities of spouses and children because they don't have as much control. They avoid lighted areas at night because they feel exposed, and they avoid dark areas anytime because the enemy can hide easily.

They also avoid big-box stores, amusement parks, farmers' markets, and other crowded places because of the fear of a suicide bomber. They drive aggressively, tailgating and refusing to yield the right of way, because that was how they survived in the Middle East. To dull their senses, numb their pain, and help them forget, they self-medicate with alcohol and rely on prescription painkillers. Some service members who return from combat are mental wrecks. Others are ticking time bombs. It doesn't help that most keep a loaded firearm near them at all times because without it they feel defenseless.

It also doesn't help that we have had an unprecedented public health crisis. On top of the stress of deploying to war zones and responding to natural disasters, during the coronavirus epidemic active-duty troops faced the same fear and uncertainty as the general public and the same sense of isolation. Welcome-home ceremonies were replaced by mandatory, two-week quarantines. Leaves were denied to service members who wanted to visit families out of state. Gyms and dining facilities on military posts closed, and in-person unit meetings were replaced by Zoom meetings. All contributed to heightened unease and reduced morale.

Early data from the first three months of 2020 indicated a slight drop in military suicides, but since then the numbers have increased significantly. By September 2020 military suicides were up 30 percent in the Army and 20 percent overall. "We cannot say definitively it [the rise in suicides] is because of Covid," Army Secretary Ryan McCarthy said, "but there is a direct correlation from when Covid started."[40]

"Covid has made us a division of strangers," Major General Christopher Donahue, commander of the 82nd Airborne Division, told reporters in September 2020. While prior to 2020 an average of four paratroopers killed themselves each year, in the first nine months of 2020 there were ten suicides in the division.[41]

What can be done? I noted a number of steps in my book *The Last and Greatest Battle*, but they can be boiled down to five.

First, all troops should be evaluated for suicide when they return home, not just those who ask for help. Evaluations should be conducted in person and one on one, not in a group with written questionnaires, as often has been the practice. In addition, evaluations should be conducted more than once to allow for delayed reactions. Family members should be interviewed as well, separately and confidentially.

Second, as much training as troops receive to prepare for battle and more needs to be provided to help them reintegrate into society when their service ends. We can't just give them pills and expect them to return to full health, as if, like tanks, they only needed a tune-up to function well again.

Third, treatment and benefits for veterans must be speeded up. Veterans shouldn't have to wait a year or more to receive health care or have their claims processed.

Fourth, the military's policy of zero tolerance when it comes to sexual harassment has to be enforced. Women in the military are twice as likely as female civilians to be raped,[42] with the assault often not reported because the victim is intimidated or afraid that it will derail her career. If it is reported, chances are good that the perpetrator—who might be a superior—will never be convicted, leading to an accuser's further depression and possible suicide attempt.

Lastly, there is the matter of stigma. The military isn't the only entity responsible for destigmatizing psychological problems that lead some people to attempt suicide, but there are steps the military can take. The most important one is to create a culture in which asking for help is accepted and not considered a weakness. More chaplains, more counselors, more accessibility, and more encouragement can foster individual well-being.

So far, the military has responded in its own way. In 2023 an independent panel recommended that the Department of Defense implement a series of gun safety measures to reduce suicides. These included waiting periods before service members can buy firearms and ammunition on military property, raising the minimum age at which service members can buy guns and ammunition to 25, and requiring anyone living in military housing to register all privately owned firearms. The panel noted that guns are used in two-thirds of all active-duty suicides and more than 70 percent of all suicides by National Guard members and reservists.[43] Already the recommendations are facing resistance in Congress and elsewhere, however, making implementation far from certain.

At least one branch of the military is making more chaplains available in an effort to reduce suicides. In the past, only the largest Navy carriers, those with five thousand or more sailors, had chaplains on board to deal with the stresses of men and women who spend most of their time below deck performing monotonous manual tasks. Today, the Navy is planning to make chaplains regular members of the crew on ships with three hundred or more sailors. The goal is for clergy to talk confidentially with both believers and nonbelievers in order to identify and treat depression. A specific challenge for Navy personnel, in addition to working in tight, windowless quarters, is that many sailors don't know life without personal phones, yet most communications are off-limits at sea for security reasons.[44] Nevertheless, any allocation of resources for this purpose is a positive step, and other branches of the military can learn from the Navy's experience.

Conclusion

When the magnitude of the task is broken down into steps like these, ending suicides no longer seems far-fetched or impossible. On the contrary, it appears doable.

"Do not go gentle into that good night," poet Dylan Thomas wrote. "Rage, rage against the dying of the light."[45] It was his way of telling people not to accept death but to fight it. In the same way, we need to rage as a society against the dying of the light in so many of our fellow citizens, neither accepting it nor ignoring the role that our apathy and ignorance play in it. It's a matter of commitment. The sooner we are willing to make it, the sooner suicides will end.

Afterword

MOST BOOKS—particularly those published by academic presses—have a long gestation period, and this book is no exception. Nearly two years will have passed between the time I submitted the final draft and *Suicide*'s publication. In the interim, some of the information has been updated, and the rest remains relevant; however, as I write this afterword in January 2024 a few recent developments are worth mentioning.

The most notable recent development is the virtual completion of the suicide-prevention net on the Golden Gate Bridge. By the latter stages of installation, the number of suicides and suicide attempts had decreased dramatically, and all indications are that going forward, the bridge no longer will be a destination for people intent on ending their lives.[1] This isn't to say that suicides from the bridge will end altogether—no solution to bridge jumps is perfect—although that is the hope. Meanwhile, advocacy continues for some sort of physical barrier—either a tall railing or a net—on other bridges with a history of suicides.[2]

Another development of note is that lawmakers continue to discuss legislative options regarding firearms. Most of these have to do with limiting the availability of rapid-fire assault weapons frequently used in mass shootings, but some reforms would make guns less accessible to suicidal individuals. The hope is that these discussions will lead to concrete actions. Each year the number of gun suicides continues to soar,[3] but most firearm suicides can be prevented with background screening of owners and responsible storage of guns and ammunition.

Another development is new data regarding CTE (chronic traumatic encephalopathy) in young contact-sports athletes. In late 2023, researchers at Boston University released their findings after examining the brains of 152 athletes younger than 30 who died by suicide. Sixty-three (41 percent) had CTE, and of this group, forty-eight played football, but no higher than the high school or college level. Other athletes in the study played hockey or soccer or wrestled.[4]

These findings led to a bill, AB 734, being introduced in California to ban tackle football for children under the age of 12. "It's not even about concussions," said the bill's author, Assemblyman Kevin McCarty. "It's about repetitive hits to the brain. If kids want to play tackle, wait until they get to puberty when their bodies are more developed."[5]

The implementation of 988 and increased funding for it and other mental health resources are positive steps in the effort to end suicides, although many people still fall through the cracks. One group that has remained largely unexamined is veterinarians. In late 2023 the BBC reported that between 1979 and 2015, nearly four hundred veterinarians in the United States died by suicide, according to data from the CDC. Male veterinarians are twice as likely to kill themselves as female veterinarians, and four times as likely as the general population. One study found that "Nearly 70 percent of veterinarians have had a colleague or peer die by suicide, and close to 60 percent have experienced work-related stress, anxiety, or depression so severe it required professional help."[6]

The reasons have to do with the nature of the job and financial factors. A key element is that animal deaths are frequent, veterinarians are trained in euthanasia procedures, and they have ready access to pentobarbital, which is one of the primary medications used for animal euthanasia. Poisoning—often with pentobarbital—is the most common cause of death among veterinarians who die by suicide. The pressure on vets to treat animals that are seriously ill and, sometimes, beyond the point of saving, weighs heavily on them, especially if pet owners can't afford costly surgery and blame vets for their pet's death. It doesn't help that the hours are long, caseloads are high, and relatively few people understand how emotionally taxing the job is. Moreover, many veterinarians have staggering debts from veterinary school. Given all of these factors, it's not surprising that their mental health suffers.

A nonprofit group, Not One More Vet, is helping veterinarians cope through an online, anonymous, peer-to-peer support program. NOMV also is raising public awareness of the problem and working to see that animal doctors pay as much attention to their own well-being as they do to that of their patients. I hope other professions learn from this model and enact similar measures.

I also hope that through this book, readers will be encouraged to pay closer attention to new studies, reports, and media stories having to do with suicide.[7] Late in 2023, the CDC reported that suicides in America in 2022 topped 49,000—a record—with elderly men at greatest risk. Meanwhile, the gender gap remained wide with over 23 deaths per 100,000 men compared with 6 per 100,000 women. Also, American Indian and Alaska Native people continued to have the highest suicide rate by race and ethnicity, nearly 27 per 100,000 people, and firearm-related suicides continued to account for more than half of all suicide deaths.[8] Clearly, the problem will not go away on its own, but with the dedication of more people, an end to this tragedy can be in sight.

Acknowledgments

Many people have educated me about suicide, mental illness, grief, and related subjects. This started with clinical staff and counselors at the Contra Costa Crisis Center, in particular Joan Stern, Judy Guthrie, Judi Hampshire, and Susan Moore. I began knowing relatively little and ended up learning a fair amount, largely because of them.

As I grew into the job, fellow executive directors at the Bay Area Suicide and Crisis Intervention Alliance (BASCIA) were an invaluable source of information, inspiration, and support. Some of them came and went, but among those who stayed I owe considerable gratitude to Ron Tauber, Eve Meyer, Janet Gorewitz, and Nancy Salamy.

On the national level, I was honored to serve on the steering committee of the National Suicide Prevention Lifeline (since renamed the 988 Suicide and Crisis Lifeline), which included many prominent and knowledgeable experts in the field of suicide prevention. Among them, John Draper, Thomas Joiner, Madelyn Gould, and Lanny Berman stood out, and I owe them more than they know.

I would be remiss if I failed to mention other members of the board of the Bridge Rail Foundation, on which I am proud to serve. Paul Muller, Dave Hull, Ken Holmes, Kay James, Dayna Whitmer, Rebecca Bernert, Richard Carlton, and Renee Amochaev each have a unique connection to suicide, yet all are committed to seeing it end.

In terms of the publication of this book, I am indebted to numerous people at Johns Hopkins University Press, starting with Joe Rusko, who was an early champion, and Suzanne Staszak-Silva, who took over after Joe left. Joanne Allen was a meticulous and masterful editor, and many others, including Charles Dibble, Diem Bloom, Kait Howard, and Kris Lykke, lent their expertise. In addition, early readers of the manuscript offered a much-needed critical review and valuable suggestions.

Last, but far from least, is my immediate family—my wife, Suzan, and our four adult children. Their encouragement and support, not only as I worked on this and other books but in my entire professional career, make everything worthwhile.

Resources

988 Suicide and Crisis Lifeline

www.988lifeline.org

Anyone who is feeling suicidal or is worried about a loved one who is suicidal can contact the Lifeline by phone or by text. It's a nonprofit organization that is based in New York City and supported by the federal government. Calls to the Lifeline are transferred seamlessly to a network of more than two hundred independent crisis centers, with callers generally connected to the center that is geographically closest to them. Licensed professionals and highly trained volunteers answer the calls 24 hours a day, 365 days a year, providing free confidential counseling and emotional support. Active-duty service members, veterans, and their families can press "1" to connect to a call center with special expertise in military issues. The Lifeline has an extensive website, plus links to every crisis center in the United States that is affiliated with it. The national, three-digit number 988 is the easiest way to access help. Other Lifeline numbers—1-800-273-TALK and 1-888-628-9454 (Spanish)—work too.

Crisis Text Line

www.crisistextline.org

Anyone in crisis can text 741741 to communicate with a trained crisis counselor. An automatic reply welcomes the texter to the service and provides a link to the organization's privacy policy. The policy notes that the person can text "STOP" at any time to end a conversation.

National Alliance on Mental Illness

www.nami.org

NAMI provides a variety of support services for mental health consumers and family members. It is a source of information on all topics related to mental illness and organizes walkathons in communities across the country to raise awareness and money for its work. Based in Virginia, the organization has local chapters in most states.

Trevor Project

www.thetrevorproject.org

Founded by the people who created *Trevor*, which won a 1995 Academy Award for short film, the Trevor Project provides crisis-intervention and suicide-prevention services to lesbian, gay, bisexual, transgender, queer, and questioning youth under the age of 25. Services include twenty-four-hour phone, text, and chat support, as well as training and research programs. 1-888-488-7386.

Training Programs

LivingWorks

www.livingworks.net

For people who seek training in suicide prevention, LivingWorks, with offices in Canada, the United States, and Australia, offers four training programs. The two primary programs are ASIST (Applied Suicide Intervention Skills Training), which lasts two full days and is conducted by two certified trainers; and safeTALK, a four-hour program. Both are open to anyone. The other two training programs are LivingWorks Start and LivingWorks Faith. For information on dates and sites of the training, contact LivingWorks or your local crisis center.

QPR Institute

www.qprinstitute.com

QPR stands for Question, Persuade, and Refer. A variety of in-person courses, ranging from three to six hours in length, teach basic skills and are open to anyone.

Suicide Prevention Resource Center

www.sprc.org

The SPRC provides in-person and online courses in suicide prevention, most of which are open to all. A few are targeted to people in behavioral health care fields. The agency also provides general information on assessing and managing suicide risk, a library of resource and training materials, and a listing of schools and tribal communities that receive suicide prevention funding from the federal Substance Abuse and Mental Health Services Administration. In addition, the SPRC maintains a best-practices registry that recognizes agencies whose suicide-prevention programs are considered to be models in the field.

Defense Suicide Prevention Office

www.dspo.mil

Established in 2011, the DSPO oversees the development, implementation, and assessment of all suicide-prevention programs, policies, and surveillance activities within the Department of Defense. Its mission, according to the official website, is to advance "holistic, data-driven suicide prevention," "positively impact individual beliefs and behaviors," and "instill systemic, cultural change" in all branches of the armed services as well as the Coast Guard.

Studies and Data

Centers for Disease Control and Prevention

www.cdc.gov

The CDC, an agency of the US Department of Health and Human Services, is responsible for protecting the health and safety of US citizens through disease control and injury prevention. In addition to providing information that aims to improve Americans' health, it engages in research projects and maintains data on suicide, other types of morbidity, disease, and injury.

National Institute of Mental Health

www.nimh.nih.gov

The NIMH, also an agency of the US Department of Health and Human Services, is the leading research institution on mental disorders. It operates twenty-seven institutes and centers that collectively make up the National Institutes of Health, considered to be the largest biomedical research agency in the world. A robust website describes its many programs and services.

American Association of Suicidology

www.suicidology.org

Although its primary focus is research, the AAS certifies crisis centers across the United States, qualifying them to handle calls from 988. Its website includes research papers, facts, statistics, and multimedia resources. The AAS also publishes a scholarly journal, *Suicide and Life-Threatening Behavior*, and hosts an annual conference that is open to the public and has separate tracks for researchers, crisis center staff, and individuals who have lost loved ones to suicide.

American Foundation for Suicide Prevention

www.afsp.org

The AFSP is the largest private funder of suicide-prevention research and services in the United States. In addition to providing grants, it promotes suicide awareness, influences public policy, provides educational and training materials, and supports families who have experienced a suicide through its Healing Conversations program.

Notes

Existence is a series of footnotes to a vast, obscure, unfinished
masterpiece.   —VLADIMIR NABOKOV

Introduction

1. Tracey, "My Son Took His Own Life."
2. Gibbs and Thompson, "War on Suicide?"
3. Jaffe, "VA Study Finds More Veterans Committing Suicide."
4. Gibbs and Thompson "War on Suicide?"
5. Khalil, "As Suicides Rise, U.S. Military Seeks to Address Mental Health."
6. Coleman, "120 War Vets Commit Suicide Each Week."
7. Coffey, "Building a System of Perfect Depression Care in Behavioral Health."
8. *Psychiatric Services*, "2006 APA Gold Award: Pursuing Perfect Depression Care."

Chapter 1. Fiction vs. Fact

1. Lester, *Making Sense of Suicide*, 29.
2. Stobbe, "U.S. Suicides Hit an All-time High Last Year."
3. Substance Abuse and Mental Health Services Administration, "Utilization of Mental Health Services by Adults with Suicidal Thoughts and Behavior."
4. Shepard et al., "Suicide and Suicidal Attempts in the United States."
5. Greenhouse, "Neglected Suicide Epidemic."

6. Rosen, "Suicide Survivors."

7. Combs, "SRJC Student Survives Jump off Golden Gate Bridge and Is Thankful at Second Chance."

8. Emanuel, "Four Myths about Doctor-Assisted Suicide."

9. Bateson, *Education of a Coroner*, 152–55.

10. Gould et al., "Evaluating Iatrogenic Risk of Youth Suicide Screening Programs."

11. Harvard T. H. Chan School of Public Health, "Means Matter: Attempters' Long-term Survival."

12. Owens, Horricks, and House, "Fatal and Non-fatal Repetition of Self-harm."

13. Bateson, *Final Leap*, 114.

14. Rafkin, "Survivor of Bridge Jump Advocates for Mental Health, Safety Barrier."

15. Qin and Nordentoft, "Suicide Risk in Relation to Psychiatric Hospitalization."

16. Hyde, "Suicide."

17. Ahmedani et al., *Racial/Ethnic Differences in Healthcare Visits Made Before Suicide Attempt across the United States.*

18. Simon et al., "Characteristics of Impulsive Suicide Attempts and Attempters."

19. Deisenhammer et al., "Duration of the Suicidal Process."

20. Barnhorst, "Empty Promises of Suicide Prevention."

21. Joiner, *Myths about Suicide*, 70.

22. Kasen, Cohen, and Chen, "Developmental Course of Impulsivity and Capability from Age 10 to Age 25."

23. Joiner, *Myths about Suicide*, 84.

24. Dubner, "Suicide Paradox."

25. Dubner.

26. Colt, *November of the Soul*, 53.

27. Colt, 54.

28. Centers for Disease Control and Prevention, "Suicide and Self-Inflicted Injury."

29. Catholic Church, *Catechism*, pt. 3, sec. 2, chap. 2, art. 5.

30. Qur'an 4:29.

31. Pew Research Center, *Muslim Publics Share Concerns about Extremist Groups.*

32. Lawrence, Oquendo, and Stanley, "Religion and Suicide Risk."

33. Hogenboom, "Many Animals Seem to Kill Themselves, but It Is Not Suicide."

34. Barbara King, quoted in Hogenboom.

35. Hogenboom.

36. Hogenboom.

37. Leenaars, "Lives and Deaths," 488.

Chapter 2. The Proverbial Question

1. Kluger, "Robin's Pain."

2. Bishop, "Search for Why."

3. Colt, *November of the Soul*, 39.

4. Menninger, *Man Against Himself*, 19.

5. Hemingway, *Nick Adams Stories*, 21.

6. Shioiri et al., "Incidence of Note-Leaving Remains Constant Despite Increasing Suicide Rates."

7. Bateson, *Final Leap*, 229–30.

8. Rabin, "Frequent Moves Increase Suicide Risk in Teens."

9. Ilgen and Kleinberg, "Link between Substance Abuse, Violence, and Suicide."

10. C. Johnson, "Sobering Report Shows Suicide Rates Rising across U.S."

11. Nutt, "Suicide Rates Rose Sharply in US, Report Shows."

12. Colt, *November of the Soul*, 41.

13. Cardinal, "Three Decades of Suicide and Life-Threatening Behavior."

14. Curwen, "His Work Is Still Full of Life."

15. Curwen.

16. *Johns Hopkins University Gazette*, "John Hopkins Team Identifies Genetic Link to Attempted Suicide."

17. ScienceDaily, "Genetic Link to Suicidal Behavior Confirmed."

18. Beck, Steer, et al., "Hopelessness and Eventual Suicide."

19. Beck, Brown, et al., "Relationship between Hopelessness and Ultimate Suicide.'"

20. Ethics of Suicide Digital Archive, "Voltaire (1694–1778), from *Philosophical Dictionary.*"

21. Joiner, *Why People Die by Suicide*, 51.

22. Bateson, *Final Leap*, 239.

23. Heyman, Dill, and Douglas, *Study: Police Officers and Firefighters Are More Likely to Die by Suicide than in the Line of Duty.*

24. Heyman, Dill, and Douglas.

25. Wild, LeBlanc, and Rose, "2 More DC Police Officers Who Responded to Capitol Insurrection Died by Suicide."

26. Joiner, *Why People Die by Suicide*, 102.

27. Hoyer and Lund, "Suicide among Women Related to Number of Children in Marriage."

28. Qin and Mortensen, "Impact of Parental Status on the Risk of Completed Suicide."

29. Tomassini et al., "Risk of Suicide in Twins."

30. Bateson, *Final Leap*, 241.

31. Joiner, *Why People Die by Suicide*, 128.

32. Levi, *Drowned and the Saved*, 76.

33. Colt, *November of the Soul*, 222.

34. Joiner, *Why People Die by Suicide*, 130–31.

35. Miller, *On Suicide*, 107.

36. Colt, *November of the Soul*, 234.

37. Colt, 238.

38. Sexton, *Complete Poems*, 142–43.

Chapter 3. By the Numbers

1. Jamison, *Night Falls Fast*, 22–23.

2. Centers for Disease Control and Prevention, "Suicide and Self-Inflicted Injury."

3. Dubner, "Suicide Paradox."

4. Archer, "White, Middle-Age Suicide in America Skyrockets."

5. Scannell, "Suicide—A Deadly Burden to Society."

6. *BBC News*, "U.S. Suicide Rate Surges, Particularly among White People."

7. Fowler et al., "Increase in Suicides Associated with Home Eviction and Foreclosure during the U.S. Housing Crisis."

8. Maugh, "Suicides and a Bad Economy Go Hand in Hand."

9. McIntosh et al., "Suicide Rates by Occupational Group—17 States, 2012."

10. Gertner, Rotter, and Shafer, "Association between State Minimum Wages and Suicide Rates in the U.S."

11. Reuters, "Higher State Minimum Wage Tied to Lower Suicide Rates."

12. Prior, "One in Four Young People Are Reporting Suicidal Thoughts."

13. Kramer, "Anxiety, Depression Mount in Bay Area."

14. Solomon, "Mystifying Rise of Child Suicide."

15. Colt, *November of the Soul*, 41.

16. Colt, 45.

17. Colt, 46.

18. Brent, Perper, and Allman, "Alcohol, Firearms, and Suicide among Youth."

19. Swaak, "How We Talk about Bullying after School Shootings Can Be Dangerous."

20. Lassne and Yanez, *Repetition and Power Imbalance in Bullying Victimization at School*.

21. Bracho-Sanchez, "Number of Children Going to ER with Suicidal Thoughts, Attempts Double, Study Finds."

22. Bracho-Sanchez, "Suicide Rates in Girls Are Rising, Study Finds, Especially in Those Age 10 to 14."

23. Colt, *November of the Soul*, 438.

24. Tanner, "Self-harm, Suicide Attempts Climb among Girls."

25. *The Week*, "Teen Suicides on the Rise."

26. Ducharme, "Almost a Third of High-School Girls Considered Suicide in 2021."

27. Suicide Prevention Resource Center, "Rate of Suicide by Race/Ethnicity, United States 2008–2017."

28. Dubner, "Suicide Paradox."

29. Conwell, Van Orden, and Caine, "Suicide in Older Adults."

30. Colt, *November of the Soul*, 256.

31. Tareen, "Pandemic, Racism Compound Worries about Black Suicide Rate."

32. Prior, "One in Four Young People Are Reporting Suicidal Thoughts."

33. Silkenat, *Moments of Despair*, 25.

34. Bateson, *Last and Greatest Battle*, 118.

35. National Humanities Center, "Suicide among Slaves."

36. Silkenat, *Moments of Despair*, 10.

37. Colt, *November of the Soul*, 260.

38. Dizmang, "Suicide among the Cheyenne Indians," 9.

39. Colt, *November of the Soul*, 260.

40. Directed by Miranda de Pencier and produced by Northwood Entertainment in Toronto, *The Grizzlies* is available on Netflix.

41. Christensen, "Living Near a Gun Shop or in a Rural Area Puts You at Higher Risk for Suicide, Study Finds."

42. Bay Area News Group, "California Gun Laws Are Helping Lower the Suicide Rate."

43. Lester and Merrell, "Influence of Gun Control Laws on Suicidal Behavior."

44. Christensen, "Living Near a Gun Shop or in a Rural Area Puts You at Higher Risk for Suicide, Study Finds."

45. Rapaport, "Suicide Rates Rising across U.S."

46. Centers for Disease Control and Prevention, "Sexual Identity, Sex of Sexual Contacts, and Health-Risk Factors among Students in Grades 9–12."

47. Assuno, "42 Percent of LGBTQ Youth Considered Suicide in 2020."

48. Garofolo et al., "Sexual Orientation and Risk of Suicide Attempts."

49. Herrel et al., "Sexual Orientation and Suicidality."

50. Colt, *November of the Soul*, 264.

51. Tanner, "Teen Suicide Attempts Higher in Conservative Area."

52. Dhejne et al., "Long-Term Follow-Up of Transsexual Persons Undergoing Sex Reassignment Surgery."

53. James et al., *Report of the 2015 U.S. Transgender Survey*.

54. Nowinski, "Troubling Trend."

55. Whyno, "Weight Watching, Injury Dangers, Caustic Feedback Add to Mental Health Woes for Horseracing Jockeys."

56. Whyno.

57. Stubbs, "After Concussions Ended Her Soccer Career, a Former Star Is Helping Girls Avoid a Similar Fate."

58. ESPN News Services, "Heather Anderson Diagnosed with CTE in 1st Case for Female Athlete."

59. Torre, "Light in the Darkness."

60. Joiner, *Why People Die by Suicide*, 130.

61. Fernquist, "Aggregate Analysis of Professional Sports, Suicide, and Homicide Rates, 30 U.S. Metropolitan Areas, 1971–1990."

62. Steels, "Deliberate Self-Poisoning."

63. Trovato, "Stanley Cup of Hockey and Suicide in Quebec, 1951–1992."

64. Lester, *Making Sense of Suicide*, 154.

65. Colt, *November of the Soul*, 250.

66. Nauert, "Majority of Suicides Occur after Midnight."

67. Kaysen, *Girl, Interrupted*, 52.

68. Falk, "Editor's Letter."

69. Dubner, "Suicide Paradox."

70. Burke et al., "Higher Temperatures Increase Suicide Rates in the United States and Mexico."

71. Burke et al.

72. Torres, "No, I'm Not 'Fine,' and There Are Millions Like Me."

73. Vitelli, "Are We Facing a Post-COVID-19 Suicide Epidemic?"

74. Clay, "COVID-19 and Suicide."

75. Hollyfield, "Suicides on the Rise amid Stay-at-Home Order, Bay Area Medical Professionals Say."

76. Reger, Stanley, and Joiner, "Suicide Mortality and Coronavirus Disease 2019—A Perfect Storm?"

77. Bartlett, "Suicide Wave That Never Was."

78. Green, "Surge of Student Suicides Pushes Las Vegas Schools to Reopen."

79. Brenner, "Report: Marin County Suicide Rate Declines."

80. Crisis Text Line, "Everybody Hurts 2020."

81. Stobbe, "U.S. Suicides Hit an All-time High Last Year."

82. McPhillips, "U.S. Suicide Rates Rose in 2021, Reversing Two Years of Decline."

83. Solomon, "Mystifying Rise of Child Suicide."

84. McPhillips, "U.S. Suicide Rates Rose in 2021, Reversing Two Years of Decline."

Chapter 4. Special Situations

1. Bateson, *Final Leap*, 109.

2. Associated Press, "National Parks Becoming Suicide Spots."

3. Centers for Disease Control and Prevention, "Suicides in National Parks."

4. Quillin, "For NC Park Rangers, Confronting Suicide Is the Worst Part of the Job."

5. Associated Press, "For Some Troubled Visitors, National Parks Become Chosen Site to End Life."

6. Gulliford, "National Parks See Suicide Upticks Each Summer."

7. Institute for Criminal Policy Research, "World Prison Brief: Highest to Lowest Prison Population Total."

8. Institute for Criminal Policy Research.

9. Towl and Crighton, *Suicide in Prisons*.

10. *San Francisco Chronicle*, "Neglect behind Prison Walls."

11. Towl and Crighton, *Suicide in Prisons*.

12. Grassian, "Psychotic Effects of Solitary Confinement."

13. Rovner, "Solitary Lockup Is Widespread and Quite Dangerous."

14. St. John, "California Suppressed Consultant's Report on Inmate Suicides."

15. *San Francisco Chronicle*, "Neglect behind Prison Walls."

16. Fagone and Cassidy, "Prison Suicides Soaring Despite Calls for Reform."

17. Fagone and Cassidy, "Prisons Chief Admits 'Suicide Crisis' after State's Report."

18. Cohen and Eckert, "Many U.S. Jails Failing to Stop Inmate Suicides."

19. National Center on Institutions and Alternatives, *National Study of Jail Suicide: 20 Years Later.*

20. Khalil, "As Suicides Rise, U.S. Military Seeks to Address Mental Health."

21. Holsworth, "Serving in Two Wars Didn't Kill Me, but the VA Might."

22. Kaplan et al., "Suicide among Male Veterans."

23. Hoge et al., "Combat Duty in Iraq and Afghanistan, Mental Health Problems, and Barriers to Care."

24. Freedman, "Tending to Veterans' Afflictions of the Soul."

25. Wilson, "Prevalence of Military Sexual Trauma."

26. Moyer, "'A Poison in the System.'"

27. Armed Forces Health Surveillance Center, "Deaths by Suicide While on Active Duty."

28. Bryan and Cukrowicz, "Associations between Types of Combat Violence and the Acquired Capability for Suicide."

29. Lubin et al., "Decrease in Suicide Rates after a Change of Policy Reducing Access to Firearms in Adolescents."

30. Harrell and Berglass, "Losing the Battle."

31. Defense Suicide Prevention Office, *CY 2022 Quarter 4 Report*, attachment A.

32. Kaufman and LeBlanc, "519 U.S. Service Members Died by Suicide in 2021, Pentagon Says."

33. Dixon-Mueller, "Last Will."

34. American Medical Association, Code of Medical Ethics, opinion 5.7.

35. Meier, "Treatment of Patients with Unbearable Suffering."

36. Worthington, "Slippery Slopes and Other Concerns."

37. Emanuel, "Whose Right to Die?"

38. *The Week*, "Spread of Assisted Suicide."

39. *The Week*, "Netherlands."

40. Associated Press, "Maine 8th State to Legalize Procedure."

41. Hutson et al., "Suicide by Cop."

42. Kucher, "Experts: 'Suicide by Cop' Cases Are Hard to Prevent."

43. Buhrmaster, "Suicide by Cop."

44. Joiner, *Perversion of Virtue*, 41.

45. Joiner, 43.

46. Colt, *November of the Soul*, 225.

47. Nock and Marzuk, "Murder-Suicide."

48. Nock and Marzuk.

Chapter 5. Talking to a Suicidal Person

1. Morris, "I Don't Want Another Family to Lose a Child the Way We Did."

2. Bateson, *Final Leap*, 149.

3. Linde, *Danger to Self*, 150.

4. Taylor, "By My Own Hand."

5. Linde, *Danger to Self*, 151.

6. Orbach, "How Would You Listen to the Person on the Roof?"

7. Shneidman, *Definition of Suicide*, 229.

8. Halderman et al., "Paradigm for the Telephonic Assessment of Suicidal Ideation."

9. Whiting, "Bernard Mayes."

10. Alonso-Zaldivar, "988 Suicide Phone Hotline Getting $282M to Ease July Launch."

11. Ramchand, Jaycox, and Ebener, "Suicide Prevention Hotlines in California."

12. Lester, *Making Sense of Suicide*, vi.

13. Gregory, "R U There?"

14. Crisis Text Line, accessed 23 November 2022, https://crisistrends.org.

15. Gregory, "R U There?"

16. Lester, *Making Sense of Suicide*, 195.

17. Giffen and Felsenthal, *A Cry for Help*, 28.

18. Colt, *November of the Soul*, 335.

19. Omer and Elitzur, "What Would You Say to the Person on the Roof?"

20. Colt, *November of the Soul*, 475.

21. *Oprah Magazine*, "Connection Cure."

22. National Suicide Prevention Lifeline, *Final Report of the Attempt Survivor Advisory Summit Meeting and Individual Interviews*, 10.

23. *Oprah Magazine*, "Best Way to Talk about Suicide."

24. *Oprah Magazine*, "Back to Life."

25. Greenhouse, "Neglected Suicide Epidemic."

26. K. Johnson, "Don't Celebrate Suicide: Educate."

27. Lester, *Making Sense of Suicide*, 168–70.

28. Hyde, "Suicide."

29. Washington State Department of Health, "Suicide Prevention Training for Health Professionals."

30. Ducharme, "Disturbing Trend on the Rise."

31. *The Week*, "Suicide."

32. Luscombe, "Things Are Never What They Seem."

33. *San Francisco Chronicle*, "Worlds We Fail to See."

34. Solomon, "Anthony Bourdain, Kate Spade, and the Preventable Tragedies of Suicide."

35. Bateson, *Final Leap*, 39.

36. Phillips, "Influence of Suggestion on Suicide."

37. Stack, "Media Coverage as a Risk Factor in Suicide."

38. Scutti, "Suicide in US Rose 10% after Robin Williams' Death, Study Finds."

39. Dubner, "Suicide Paradox."

40. Niederkrotenthaler, "Role of Media Reports in Completed and Prevented Suicide."

41. Lester, *Making Sense of Suicide*, 148.

42. Jamieson, Jamieson, and Romer, "Can Suicide Coverage Lead to Copycats?"

Chapter 6. Guns and Suicide

1. Agresti and Smith, "Gun Control Facts."

2. Kounang, "America's Doctors Call for Strongest Gun Control Measures to Date."

3. *Personal Defense World*, "Small Arms Survey."

4. Elliott, Edwards, and Alter, "After the Massacre."

5. Drexler, "Guns and Suicide."

6. Elliott, Edwards, and Alter, "After the Massacre."

7. Cillizza, "8 Charts That Explain America's Gun Culture."

8. Colt, *November of the Soul*, 348.

9. Echeverria, "Suicide Likelier for Women in Homes with Gun."

10. Asimov, "Stanford study."

11. Miller and Hemenway, "Guns and Suicide in the United States."

12. *The Week*, "Noted."

13. Davis, *Don't Know Much About History*, 85.

14. Erdozain, "What the Founding Fathers Would Say about Mass Shootings."

15. Mann et al., "Suicide Prevention Strategies."

16. Giffords Law Center to Prevent Gun Violence, "Truth about Guns and Suicide."

17. Drexler, "Guns and Suicide."

18. Harvard T. H. Chan School of Public Health, "Means Matter: Firearm Access Is a Risk Factor for Suicide."

19. Centers for Disease Control and Prevention, "Suicide by Method." n

20. Drexler, "Guns and Suicide."

21. Johns Hopkins Bloomberg School of Public Health, "CDC Provisional Data: Gun Suicides Reach All-time High in 2022."

22. Johns Hopkins Bloomberg School of Public Health.

23. Johns Hopkins Bloomberg School of Public Health.

24. Harvard T. H. Chan School of Public Health, "Means Matter: Firearm Access Is a Risk Factor for Suicide."

25. Miller and Hemenway, "Guns and Suicide in the United States."

26. Drexler, "Guns and Suicide."

27. Peck and Fox, "To Reduce Risk of Mass Shootings, Help Prevent Suicides."

28. Gilmour and Tehee, "Why Toy Guns—but Not Real Guns—Are Banned on the Las Vegas Strip."

29. Wills, "Spiking the Gun Myth."

30. Wills.

31. Colt, *November of the Soul*, 347.

32. Cillizza, "8 Charts That Explain American's Gun Culture."

33. *The Week*, "Armed and Dangerous," 11.

34. First reported by German Lopez on Vox.com and cited by *The Week* in "A Gunman's Deadly Rampage in a Texas Church," 5.

35. *The Week*, "Armed and Dangerous," 11.

36. *The Week*, "Rise of White Supremacist Terrorism."

37. Onyanga-Omara, "Gun Violence Rare in U.K. Compared to U.S."

38. Onyanga-Omara.

39. *The Week*, "Armed and Dangerous," 11.

40. Gold and Ramsey, "It's Not about Linking Gun Violence and Mental Illness."

41. *The Week*, "Video Games and Violence."

42. *The Week*, "Guns."

43. Sorkin, "Guns and the City."

44. Bergen, "America the Lethal."

45. Healy, "The Stronger a State's Gun Laws, the Lower Its Rate of Gun-Related Homicides and Suicides."

46. *The Week*, "Newtown, Conn., and Parkland, Fla. Horrors Persist."

47. McQueen, "Twenty Years after That Day at Columbine High School."

48. Tanner, "Half of Fatalities Come from 6 Nations, Including U.S."

49. Elliott, Edwards, and Alter, "After the Massacre."

50. Cillizza, "8 Charts That Explain American's Gun Culture."

51. Abrams and Chan, "Special Report: Guns in America."

52. Elliott, Edwards, and Alter, "After the Massacre."

53. Giffords Law Center to Prevent Gun Violence, "Universal Background Checks."

54. Andelman, "How France Cut Its Per Capita Gun Ownership in Half."

55. Alliance Vita, *Suicide in France: Third Official Report*.

56. J. Lee, "What We Can Learn from Canada on Gun Control."

57. Grossman et al., "Gun Storage Practices and Risk of Youth Suicide and Unintentional Firearm Injuries."

58. Giffords Law Center to Prevent Gun Violence, "Truth about Guns and Suicide."

59. Healy, "The Stronger a State's Gun Laws, the Lower Its Rate of Gun-Related Homicide and Suicides."

60. Drexler, "Guns and Suicide."

61. Harrell and Berglass, "Losing the Battle."

62. Phillipps, "Issue of Firearms Hinders Veterans' Suicide Prevention."

63. Dwyer, "If Guns Do Not Kill, Tax the Bullets."

64. Gelles, "Why Not Tax Bullets?"

65. Drexler, "Guns and Suicide."

66. John Draper, email to members of board of directors, Bridge Rail Foundation, 21 November 2017.

67. Shute, "Plan to Prevent Gun Suicides."

68. Shute.

69. Daley, "State, Doctors Get Welcome Allies."

70. Zoellner, "Gun Industry's Takeover Silences Group's Suicide Prevention Message."

71. Dunkerly, "Gun Lobby Is Hindering Suicide Prevention."

72. American Foundation for Suicide Prevention, "AFSP's Position on Firearms and Suicide Prevention."

73. Robert Gebbia, letter to the editor, sent to the *New York Times* and other papers, emailed to author by Stephanie Rogers, senior vice president, Communications and Marketing, AFSP, 7 January 2022.

73. *The Week*, "Armed and Dangerous."

74. Satia, "Mass Shootings and the Arms Industry."

Chapter 7. Drugs and Suicide

1. Hass et al., *American Poetry: The Twentieth Century*, 1:871.

2. Colt, *November of the Soul*, 399.

3. Colt.

4. Ross, "Suicide: One of Addiction's Hidden Risks."

5. Ilgen and Kleinberg, "Link between Substance Abuse, Violence, and Suicide."

6. Goodnough, Sanger-Katz, and Katz, "Drug Overdose Deaths Drop in US for First Time since 1990."

7. Erdman, "Drug Overdose Deaths Jump in 2019 to Nearly 70,000, a Record High, CDC Says."

8. Associated Press, "U.S. Overdose Deaths Hit Record 93,000 in Pandemic Last Year."

9. Centers for Disease Control and Prevention, "Drug Overdose Deaths Remained High in 2921."

10. National Center for Health Statistics, "Provisional Data Shows U.S. Drug Overdose Deaths Top 100,000 in 2022."

11. Buckley and Eddleston, "Paracetamol (Acetaminophen) Poisoning."

12. Mann et al., "Suicide Prevention Strategies."

13. Colt, *November of the Soul*, 318.

14. Colt, 322.

15. Colt, 321.

16. Sapatkin, "Suicides Involving Opioids More than Doubled in 15 Years, Study Finds."

17. D. Simon, "Opioid Epidemic Is So Bad That Librarians Are Learning How to Treat Overdoses."

18. Uquendo, "Opioid Use Disorders and Suicide."

19. Uquendo and Volkow, "Suicide: A Silent Contributor to Opioid-Overdose Deaths."

20. Ashrafioun et al., "Frequency of Prescription Opioid Use and Suicidal Ideation, Planning, and Attempts."

21. Leinwand Leger, "OxyContin a Gateway to Heroin for Upper-Income Addicts."

22. Rosenberg, "How One Town Got Hooked."

23. Leinwand Leger, "OxyContin a Gateway to Heroin for Upper-Income Addicts."

24. Calabresi, "Price of Relief."

25. Erdman, "Drug Overdose Deaths Jump in 2019 to Nearly 71,000, a Record High, CDC Says."

26. National Center for Health Statistics, "U.S. Overdose Deaths in 2021 Increased Half as Much as in 2020."

27. National Center for Health Statistics.

28. Associated Press, "Overdose Deaths Higher in Cities Than Rural Areas."

29. Moakley, "Eight Questions."

30. *Los Angeles Times*, "Fatal Overdoses Drop after Crackdown on Pill Mills."

31. *New York Times*, "Inside a Killer Drug Epidemic."

32. Edwards, "Drug Cascade."

33. Gelineau, "Opioid Addiction on Rise in Sad Echo of U.S. Crisis."

34. Daly, *Generation Rx*, 1.

Chapter 8. Jump Sites and Suicide

1. Olson, "'Jumping' and Suicide Prevention."

2. Draper, "Suicide Prevention on Bridges."

3. New York State Bridge Authority, *Comprehensive Plan for Suicide Prevention*.

4. Draper, "Suicide Prevention on Bridges."

5. Draper.

6. Donaldson, "Suicide Bridge Reduces Impulse to Jump."

7. Calder, "Barrier Proposed to Prevent Verrazzano Bridge Suicides."

8. Dotinga, "One Year In, 'Bird Spikes' Haven't Stopped Coronado Bridge Suicides."

9. J. Jones, "Skyway Safeguards Don't Deter Jumpers."

10. Marrero, "Sunshine Skyway Bridge to Get Suicide Prevention Barrier."

11. Sinyor and Levitt, "Effect of a Barrier at Bloor Street Viaduct on Suicide Rates in Toronto."

12. Bateson, *Final Leap*, 196–97.

13. Beautrais, "Suicide by Jumping."

14. Bennewith, Nowers, and Gunnell, "Effect of Barriers on the Clifton Suspension Bridge, England, on Local Patterns of Suicide."

15. Stephens, "Golden Gate Follows Bern's Lead with Suicide Nets."

16. Pelletier, "Preventing Suicide by Jumping."

17. Bateson, *Final Leap*, 202.

18. Rivera, "Temporary Suicide Prevention Fencing Cuts Fatalities at Colorado Street Bridge."

19. Rilkoff, Sanford, and Fordham, *Interventions to Prevent Suicide from Bridges*, 27.

20. Rilkoff, Sanford, and Fordham, 3.

21. O'Neill, "Dark History of Beautiful Spots Where Hundreds Have Died."

22. Norrie, "New Fence at The Gap 'Just Not High Enough.'"

23. Maynard, "Australia Mourns 'Angel of the Gap' Don Ritchie."

24. Gelineau, "Australian 'Angel' Saves Lives at Suicide Spot."

25. Norrie, "New Fence at The Gap 'Just Not High Enough.'"

26. California Department of Mental Health. *California Strategic Plan on Suicide Prevention*, 22.

27. Stanford Suicide Prevention Research Lab, *Novel Therapeutics for Suicide Prevention*.

28. Aitkens et al., *Guidance on Action to Be Taken at Suicide Hotspots*.

29. Wang, Wright, and Wakatsuki, "In Japan, More People Died from Suicide Last Month than from Covid in All of 2020."

30. Kaiman, "At Japan's Suicide Cliffs, He's Walked More than 600 People Back from the Edge."

31. MacFarquhar, "Last Call."

32. See www.atlasobscura.com.

33. DeMarco, "Glamorize Death and Copycat Suicides Follow."

34. Kaiman, "At Japan's Suicide Cliffs, He's Walked More than 600 People Back from the Edge."

35. Wang, Wright, and Wakatsuki, "In Japan, More People Died from Suicide Last Month than from Covid in All of 2020."

36. Rosin, "Silicon Valley Suicides."

37. Yuasa, "With Suicides a Concern, Japan Tries Mood Lights."

38. Matasubayashi, Sawada, and Ueda, "Does the Installation of Blue Lights on Train Platforms Shift Suicide to Another Station? Evidence from Japan."

39. Matasubayashi, Sawada, and Ueda, "Does the Installation of Blue Lights on Train Platforms Prevent Suicide? A Before-and-after Observational Study from Japan."

40. New.com.au, "Train Suicides Spike after Rain in Japan."

41. Yuasa, "With Suicides a Concern, Japan Tries Mood Lights."

42. Richarz, "Amazing Psychology of Japanese Train Stations."

Chapter 9. Success Story

1. These and other annual statistics cited in this chapter are from Golden Gate Bridge, Highway, and Transportation District, *GGBHTD Incident Reports Relative to Suicide by Calendar Year.*

2. V. Ho, "Golden Gate Bridge Suicides Hit Record High—46."

3. Prado, "Family Struggles with Death of Teen Son from Golden Gate Bridge."

4. L. Johnson, "Finding Kyle."

5. Koopman, "No Easy Death."

6. Bateson, *Final Leap*, 82.

7. Bateson, 97.

8. Bateson, 145.

9. Nevius, "Taking a Little Time to Listen Could Save a Life."

10. Marin County Coroner's Office and the Bridge Rail Foundation, *Fifteen-Year Report: Golden Gate Bridge Suicide Demographics.*

11. Jerry Check, email correspondence with author, February 2023.

12. Koopman, "No Easy Death."

13. Ken Holmes, email correspondence with author, February 2023.

14. Kreitman, "Coal Gas Story."

15. Seiden, "Where Are They Now?"

16. Seiden and Spence, "Tale of Two Bridges."

17. Brown, *Golden Gate*, 201.

18. Friend, "A Net, at Last, for the Golden Gate Bridge?"

Chapter 10. Ending Suicide

1. Dubner, "Suicide Paradox."

2. Dubner.

3. *Economist*, "Why Suicide Is Falling around the World."

4. Tanner, "Rise in Suicide and Social Media Coincide."

5. Coffey, "Pursuing Perfect Depression Care: A Model for Eliminating Suicide and Transforming Mental Healthcare."

6. Seyrig, "Depression Care Program Eliminates Suicide."

7. Coffey, "Building a System of Perfect Depression Care in Behavioral Health."

8. *Psychiatric Services*, "2006 APA Gold Award: Pursuing Perfect Depression Care."

9. zerosuicide.edc.org.

10. Layman et al., "Relationship between Suicidal Behaviors and Zero Suicide Organizational Best Practices in Outpatient Mental Health Clinics."

11. *Psychiatric News*, "'Zero Suicide' Practices at Mental Health Clinics Reduce Suicide among Patients, Study Finds."

12. Stapelberg et al., "Efficacy of the Zero Suicide Framework in Reducing Recurrent Suicide Attempts."

13. Moriki, "Exhibit Seeks to Stop Suicide."

14. Campbell, "She Lost Too Many Friends to Suicide."

15. Elassar, "Son of an Iraq War Veteran Designed an App to Stop His Dad's PTSD Nightmares."

16. Austin, "I Was a Pastor When I Nearly Died by Suicide."

17. Echeverria and Newcomb, "'What Am I Doing Wrong?'"

18. Wong and Gold, "Fourth Suicide at the Vessel Leads to Calls for Higher Barrier."

19. Schulman, "Healing Together."

20. D. Williams, "Wisconsin Farmers Turned Their Corn Maze into an 11-Acre Billboard for a Suicide Helpline."

21. Whiting, "Resource of Hope for Mental Healing."

22. Romo, "Truckers Line Up under Bridge to Save Man Threatening Suicide."

23. *East Bay Times*, "Bay Area County's Suicide Prevention Efforts Are Working."

24. Holmes, "Suicide Deterrent Construction on Coronado Bridge to Start in 4 Years."

25. *Santa Fe New Mexican*, "Our View: Safety at the Gorge Bridge Has Been Neglected Too Long."

26. Wan, "Chesapeake Bay Bridge Suicides."

27. Bengal, "Officials Prioritize Curbing Astoria Bridge Suicides."

28. Barrett, "Lawmakers Want Barriers Erected on Three Newport County Bridges to Deter Suicide Attempts."

29. Fitzpatrick, "Advocates Question Why Newport Pell Bridge Funding Did Not Include Suicide Barriers."

30. Ola, "Hoan Bridge New Safety Measure Seen as Potentially Life-Saving"; Adolpjus, "NY Bridge Safety Summit Eyes Suicide Prevention Measures"; *ABC Fox News Montana*, "Spokane City Council and Fire Officials Pushing for Protective Barriers on Monroe St. Bridge."

31. Bandara et al., "Cost-Effectiveness of Installing Barriers at Bridge and Cliff Sites for Suicide Prevention in Australia."

32. Miller and Hemenway, "Relationship between Firearms and Suicide."

33. Peck and Fox, "To Reduce Risk of Mass Shootings, Help Prevent Suicides."

34. An act to authorize funds for Federal-aid highways, highway safety programs, and transit programs, and for other purposes, Public Law 112-141 (6 July 2012), §§ 1108(a)(7) and 1101(1).

35. Augusta Free Press, "Legislation Aimed at Reducing Suicide Attempts at Bridges Introduced in Congress."

36. Morales and Almasy, "NYPD Officer Has Died by Suicide."

37. Law, "New York City Police Officer Dies by Suicide."

38. Perry, "Grim Exit Lines Gathered into Book."

39. Law, "New York City Police Officer Dies by Suicide."

40. Baldor and Burns, "Military Suicides Up 20% amid Host of Challenges."

41. Morgan, "As Suicides Rise, Army Brass Reassessing Outreach."

42. Benedict, "Why Soldiers Rape."

43. Associated Press, "Panel: Military Needs Gun Safety Measures to Limit Suicides."

44. Associated Press, "U.S. Navy Deploys More Chaplains for Suicide Prevention."

45. Thomas, *Poems of Dylan Thomas*, 239.

Afterword

1. Branch, "What the Golden Gate Is (Finally) Doing About Suicides."

2. Mullen, Walton, and McGrory, "Opinion: An Inexpensive Barbwire Barrier Could Stop the Coronado Bridge Suicides."

3. McPhillips, "With Gun Suicides at Record Levels in the U.S., Rates Differ Markedly by State Policies on Gun Safety."

4. Bracken, Branch, Laffin, Lieberman, and Ward, [Interactive] "They Started Playing Football as Young as 6; They Died in Their Teens and Twenties with C.T.E."

5. Haubner. "New California Bill Aims to Ban Tackle Football for Kids 12 and Under."

6. K. Morgan, "Acute Suicide Crisis Among Veterinarians."

7. Lezra, "A Stranger Asked Me to Take Her Photograph."

8. Reyes, "Suicides in U.S. Hit Historic High in 2022."

Bibliography

Books

Alvarez, A. *The Savage God: A Study of Suicide.* New York: W. W. Norton, 1971.

Bateson, John. *The Education of a Coroner: Lessons in Investigating Death.* New York: Scribner, 2017.

_____. *The Final Leap: Suicide on the Golden Gate Bridge.* Berkeley: University of California Press, 2012.

_____. *The Last and Greatest Battle: Finding the Will, Commitment, and Strategy to End Military Suicides.* New York: Oxford University Press, 2015.

Bellesiles, Michael A. *Arming America: The Origins of a National Gun Culture.* New York: Knopf, 2000.

Berman, Alan L., David A. Jobes, and Morton M. Silverman. *Adolescent Suicide: Assessment and Intervention.* Washington, DC: American Psychological Association, 2006.

Bolton, Iris. *My Son . . . My Son . . . : A Guide to Healing After Death, Loss, or Suicide.* With Curtis Mitchell. Rev. ed. Atlanta: Bolton Press, 1993.

Brown, Allen. *Golden Gate: Biography of a Bridge.* New York: Doubleday, 1965.

Carlson, Richard James. *I'm in the Tub, Gone.* Baltimore: Publish America, 2004.

Colt, George Howe. *November of the Soul: The Enigma of Suicide.* New York: Scribner, 2006.

Daly, Erin Marie. *Generation Rx: A Story of Dope, Death, and America's Opiate Crisis.* Berkeley, CA: Counterpoint, 2014.

Davis, Kenneth C. *Don't Know Much About History: Everything You Need to Know about American History but Never Learned.* New York: Crown, 1990.

Durkheim, Émile. *Suicide.* New York: Free Press, 1951.

Fedden, H. R. *Suicide: A Social and Historical Study.* New York: Benjamin Blim, 1972.

Giffen, Mary Elizabeth, and Carol Felsenthal. *A Cry for Help.* New York: Knopf, 1983.

Grossman, Dave. *On Killing: The Psychological Cost of Learning to Kill in War and Society.* New York: Back Bay Books, 2009.

Hass, Robert, John Hollander, Carolyn Kizer, Nathaniel Mackey, and Marjorie Perloff, comps. *American Poetry: The Twentieth Century.* Volume 1, *Henry Adams to Dorothy Parker.* New York: Library of America, 2000.

Heckler, Richard A. *Waking Up, Alive.* New York: Ballantine Books, 1994.

Hemingway, Ernest. *The Nick Adams Stories.* New York: Scribner, 2009.

Humphrey, Derek. *Final Exit: The Practicalities of Self-Deliverance and Assisted Suicide for the Dying.* New York: Dell, 2002.

Hunt, Tom. *Cliffs of Despair: A Journey to the Edge.* New York: Random House, 2007.

Jamison, Kay Redfield. *Night Falls Fast: Understanding Suicide.* New York: Knopf, 1999.

_____. *An Unquiet Mind.* New York: Knopf, 1995.

Jobes, David A. *Managing Suicidal Risk: A Collaborative Approach.* New York: Guilford, 2006.

Joiner, Thomas. *Myths about Suicide.* Cambridge, MA: Harvard University Press, 2010.

_____. *The Perversion of Virtue: Understanding Murder-Suicide.* New York: Oxford University Press, 2014.

_____. *Why People Die by Suicide.* Cambridge, MA: Harvard University Press, 2005.

Kadison, Richard, and Theresa Foy Digeronimo. *College of the Overwhelmed: The Campus Mental Health Crisis and What to Do about It.* San Francisco: Josey-Bass, 2004.

Kaysen, Susanna. *Girl, Interrupted.* New York: Vintage, 1994.

Kutchins, Herb, and Stuart A. Kirk. *Making Us Crazy: DSM; The Psychiatric Bible and the Creation of Mental Illness.* New York: Simon & Schuster, 1997.

Lester, David. *Crisis Intervention and Counseling by Telephone and the Internet*. 3rd ed. Springfield, IL: Charles C. Thomas, 2012

———. *Making Sense of Suicide: An In-depth Look at Why People Kill Themselves*. Philadelphia: Charles Press, 1997.

Levi, Primo. *The Drowned and the Saved*. Reissue. New York: Simon & Schuster, 2017.

Linde, Paul R. *Danger to Self: On the Front Line with an ER Psychiatrist*. Berkeley: University of California Press, 2010.

MacDonald, Donald, and Ira Nadel. *Golden Gate Bridge: History and Design of an Icon*. San Francisco: Chronicle Books, 2008.

Macy, Beth. *Dopesick: Dealers, Doctors, and the Drug Company That Addicted America*. Boston: Little, Brown, 2018.

Marcus, Eric. *Why Suicide?* New York: HarperCollins, 2010.

Menninger, Karl. *Man Against Himself*. New York: Harcourt Brace, 1938.

Miller, John, ed. *On Suicide: Great Writers on the Ultimate Question*. San Francisco: Chronicle Books, 1992.

Quinnett, Paul G. *Suicide: The Forever Decision*. New York: Continuum, 1992.

Sexton, Anne. *The Complete Poems*. New York: Ecco, 1999.

Shea, Shawn C. *The Practical Art of Suicide Assessment*. Hoboken, NJ: John Wiley & Sons, 2002.

Shneidman, Edwin S. *Autopsy of a Suicidal Mind*. New York: Oxford University Press, 2004.

———. *A Commonsense Book of Death*. Lanham, MD: Rowman & Littlefield, 2009.

———. *Definition of Suicide*. New York: Regina Ryan, 1983.

———. *The Suicidal Mind*. New York: Oxford University Press, 1996.

Silkenat, David. *Moments of Despair: Suicide, Divorce, and Debt in Civil War North Carolina*. Chapel Hill: University of North Carolina Press, 2011.

Starr, Kevin. *Golden Gate: The Life and Times of America's Greatest Bridge*. New York: Bloomsbury, 2010.

Styron, William. *Darkness Invisible: A Memoir of Madness*. New York: Vintage, 1992.

Thomas, Dylan. *The Poems of Dylan Thomas*. New York: New Directions, 2003.

Van der Zee, John. *The Gate: The True Story of the Design and Construction of the Golden Gate Bridge*. New York: Simon & Schuster, 2000.

Yalom, Irvin D. *The Gift of Therapy: An Open Letter to a New Generation of Therapists and Their Patients*. New York: HarperCollins, 2002.

Studies and Reports

Ahmedani, B. K., Christine Stewart, Gregory E. Simon, et al. *Racial Differences in Healthcare Visits Made Prior to Suicide Attempt across the United States*. National Institutes of Health, 2015.

Aitkens, Peter, Christabel Owens, Sally Lloyd-Tomlins, et al. *Guidance on Action to Be Taken at Suicide Hotspots*. National Institute for Mental Health in England, October 2006.

Alliance Vita. *Suicide in France: Third Official Report*. 16 February 2018.

American College Health Association. *National College Health Assessment: Reference Group Report*. 2002.

Armed Forces Health Surveillance Center. "Deaths by Suicide While on Active Duty, Active and Reserve Components, U.S. Armed Forces, 1998–2011." *Medical Surveillance Monthly Report*, June 2012.

Ashrafioun, Lisham, Todd Bishop, Kenneth Conner, et al. "Frequency of Prescription Opioid Use and Suicidal Ideation, Planning, and Attempts." *Journal of Psychiatric Research* 92 (September 2017): 1–7.

Bandara, Plumee, Jane Pirkis, Angela Clapperton, et al. "Cost-Effectiveness of Installing Barriers at Bridges and Cliff Sites for Suicide Prevention in Australia." *JAMA Network Open* 5, no. 4 (April 2022): 3226019.

Beautrais, Annette L. "Effectiveness of Barriers at Suicide Jumping Sites: A Case Study." *Australian and New Zealand Journal of Psychiatry* 35, no. 5 (2001).

———. "Suicide by Jumping: A Review of Research on Prevention Strategies." *Crisis: The Journal of Crisis Intervention and Suicide Prevention* 28, suppl. 1 (January 2007): 58–63.

Beautrais, A. L., S. D. Gibb, L. J. Horwood, and G. L. Larkin. "Removing Bridge Barriers Stimulates Suicides." *Australian and New Zealand Journal of Psychiatry* 43, no. 6 (June 2009): 495–97.

Beck, Aaron T., Gary Brown, Robert J. Berchick, et al. "Relationship between Hopelessness and Ultimate Suicide: A Replication with Psychiatric Outpatients." *Focus: The Journal of Lifelong Learning in Psychiatry* 4, no. 2 (April 2006).

Beck, A. T., M. Kovacs, and A. Weissman. "Hopelessness and Suicidal Behavior." *JAMA* 234, no. 11 (December 1975): 1146–49.

Beck, A. T., R. A. Steer, and M. G. Carbin. "Psychometric Properties of the Beck Depression Inventory: Twenty-five Years of Evaluation." *Clinical Psychology Review* 8, no. 1 (1988): 77–100.

Beck, A. T., R. A. Steer, M. Kovacs, and B. Garrison. "Hopelessness and Eventual Suicide: A 10-Year Prospective Study of Patients Hospitalized with Suicidal Ideation." *American Journal of Psychiatry* 142, no. 5 (May 1985): 559–63.

Bennewith, O., M. Nowers, and D. Gunnell. "Effect of Barriers on the Clifton Suspension Bridge, England, on Local Patterns of Suicide: Implications for Prevention." *British Journal of Psychiatry* 190 (2007): 266–67.

Bickley, Harriet, Lisabelle M. Hunt, Kirsten Windfuhr, et al. "Suicide within Two Weeks of Discharge from Psychiatric Inpatient Care: A Case-Control Study." *Psychiatric Services* 64, no. 7 (July 2013): 653–59.

Blaustein, M., and A. Fleming. "Suicide from the Golden Gate Bridge." *American Journal of Psychiatry* 166, no. 10 (October 2009): 1111–16.

Breggin, P. R. "Suicidality, Violence, and Mania Caused by Selective Serotonin Reuptake Inhibitors (SSRIs)." *Internal Journal of Risk and Safety in Medicine* 16, no. 1 (2003): 31–49.

Brent, D. A., J. A. Perper, and C. J. Allman. "Alcohol, Firearms, and Suicide among Youth: Temporal Trends in Allegheny County, Pennsylvania, 1960 to 1983." *JAMA* 257, no. 24 (1987): 3369–72.

Bryan, Craig J., and Kelly C. Cukrowicz. "Associations between Types of Combat Violence and the Acquired Capability for Suicide." *Suicide and Life-Threatening Behavior* 41, no. 2 (April 2011): 126–36.

Buckley, Nick, and Michael Eddleston. "Paracetamol (Acetaminophen) Poisoning." *British Medical Journal*, December 2007, 2101.

Burke, Marshall, Felipe González, Patrick Baylis, et al. "Higher Temperatures Increase Suicide Rates in the United States and Mexico." *Nature Climate Change*, July 2018.

California Department of Mental Health. *California Strategic Plan on Suicide Prevention: Every Californian Is Part of the Solution*. Sacramento, 2008.

Callanan, V. J., and M. S. Davis. "A Comparison of Suicide Note Writers with Suicides Who Did Not Leave Notes." *Suicide and Life-Threatening Behavior* 39, no. 5 (October 2009): 558–68.

Cantor, C. H., and M. A. Hill. "Suicide from River Bridges." *Australian and New Zealand Journal of Psychiatry* 24, no. 3 (September 1990): 377–80.

Carbone, Jason T., Katherine J. Holzer, and Michael G. Vaughn. "Child and Adolescent Suicidal Ideation and Suicide Attempts: Evidence from the Healthcare Cost and Utilization Project." *Journal of Pediatrics* 206 (March 2019): 225–31.

Cardinal, Charles. "Three Decades of Suicide and Life-Threatening Behavior: A Bibliometric Study." *Suicide and Life-Threatening Behavior* 38, no. 3 (June 2008): 260–73.

Centers for Disease Control and Prevention. "Drug Overdose Deaths Remained High in 2021." 10 August 2022.

————. "Sexual Identity, Sex of Sexual Contacts, and Health-Risk Factors among Students in Grades 9–12." *Morbidity and Mortality Weekly Report* 65, no. 9 (12 August 2016).

————. "Suicides in National Parks—United States, 2003–2009." *Morbidity and Mortality Weekly Report* 59, no. 47 (3 December 2010): 1546–49.

Clay, Rebecca A. "COVID-19 and Suicide: How the Pandemic Will Affect Suicide Rates Is Still Unknown, But There's Much Psychologists Can Do to Mitigate Its Impact." Covid-19 Special Report. American Psychological Association, 1 June 2020. https://www.apa.org/monitor/2020/06/covid-suicide.

Coffey, C. Edward. "Building a System of Perfect Depression Care in Behavioral Health." *Joint Commission Journal on Quality and Safety* 33, no. 4 (April 2007): 193–99.

————. "Pursuing Perfect Depression Care." *Psychiatric Services* 57, no. 10 (October 2006): 1524–26.

Conwell, Yeates, Kimberly Van Orden, and Eric D. Caine. "Suicide in Older Adults." *Psychiatric Clinics of North America* 34, no. 2 (June 2011): 451–68.

Crisis Text Line. "Everybody Hurts 2020." www.crisistextline.org.

Curwen, T. "His Work Is Still Full of Life." *Los Angeles Times*, 5 June 2004.

Daigle, M. S. "Suicide Prevention through Means Restriction: Assessing the Risk of Substitution." *Accident Analysis and Prevention* 37 (2005): 625–32.

Davidson, C. L., L. R. Wingate, K. A. Rasmussen, and M. L. Slish. "Hope as a Predictor of Interpersonal Suicide Risk." *Suicide and Life-Threatening Behavior* 39, no. 5 (October 2009): 499–507.

Defense Suicide Prevention Office. *CY 2022 Quarter 4 Report*. Attachment A. Accessed 16 August 2023. https://www.dspo.mil/Portals/113/Documents/2022QSR/TAB%20A%20-%20QSR%20Rpt_Q4%20CY22_vf.pdf?ver=oLwAC6aBdl1Kc58EvKk6Uw%3D%3D.

Deisenhammer, E. A., C. M. Ing, R. Strauss, et al. "The Duration of the Suicidal Process: How Much Time Is Left for Intervention between Consideration and Accomplishment of a Suicide Attempt?" *Journal of Clinical Psychiatry* 70, no. 1 (January 2009): 19–24.

Dhejne, Cecilia, Paul Lichtenstein, Marcus Boman, et al. "Long-Term Follow-up of Transsexual Persons Undergoing Sex Reassignment Surgery: Cohort Study in Sweden." *PLoS/One* 6, no. 2 (2011): e16885.

Dizmang, L. H. "Suicide among the Cheyenne Indians." *Bulletin of Suicidology* 1 (July 1967): 8–11.

Draper, John. "Suicide Prevention on Bridges: The National Suicide Prevention Lifeline Position." National Suicide Prevention Lifeline. Revised January 2017.

Drexler, Madeline. "Guns and Suicide: The Hidden Toll." *Harvard Public Health*, Spring 2013, 24–40.

Ethics of Suicide Digital Archive. "Voltaire (1694–1778), from *Philosophical Dictionary.*" 23 May 2015.

Ezzell, Carol. "Why? The Neuroscience of Suicide." *Scientific American* 288, no. 2 (February 2003): 44–51.

Fernquist, R. M. "An Aggregate Analysis of Professional Sports, Suicide, and Homicide Rates, 30 U.S. Metropolitan Areas, 1971–1990." *Aggression and Violent Behavior* 5, no. 4 (2000): 329–41.

Florentine, J. B., and C. Crane. "Suicide Prevention by Limiting Access to Means: A Review of Theory and Practice." *Social Science & Medicine* 70, no, 10 (May 2010): 1626–32.

Fowler, Katherine A., R. Matthew Gladden, Kevin J. Vagi, et al. "Increase in Suicides Associated with Home Eviction and Foreclosure during the US Housing Crisis: Findings from 16 National Violent Death reporting System States: 2005–1010," *American Journal of Public Health* 105, no. 2 (February 2015): 311–16.

Garofolo, Robert, R. Cameron Wolf, Lawrence S. Wissow, at al. "Sexual Orientation and Risk of Suicide Attempts among a Representative Sample of Youth," *Archives of Pediatrics and Adolescent Medicine* 153 (1999): 487–93.

Gertner, Alex K., Jason S. Rotter, and Paul R. Shafer. "Association between State Minimum Wages and Suicide Rates in the U.S." *American Journal of Preventive Medicine* 56, no. 5 (May 2019): 648–54.

Golden Gate Bridge, Highway, and Transportation District. *GGBHTD Incident Reports Relative to Suicide by Calendar Year.* Report received via email 4 January 2022.

———. *Suicide Deterrent System (SDS) Information.* Distributed to the media 16 May 2019. www.goldengatebridgenet.org.

Gould, Madelyn S., Frank A. Marrocco, Marjorie Kleinman, et al. "Evaluating Iatrogenic Risk of Youth Suicide Screening Programs: A Randomized Controlled Trial." *JAMA* 293, no. 13 (April 2005): 1635–43.

Grassian, Stuart. "Psychotic Effects of Solitary Confinement." *Washington University Journal of Law and Policy* 22, no. 1 (January 2006).

Grossman, David C., Beth A. Mueller, Christine A. Riedy, et al. "Gun Storage Practices and Risk of Youth Suicide and Unintentional Firearm Injuries," *JAMA* 293, no. 60 (2005): 707–14.

Grunbaum, Jo Ann, Laura Kann, Steven A. Kinchen, et al. "2001 Youth Risk Behavior Surveillance." *Morbidity and Mortality Weekly Report* 5, no. 4 (28 June 2002): 1–62.

Halderman, Brent L., James R. Eyman, Lisa Kerner, and Bill Schlacks. "A Paradigm for the Telephonic Assessment of Suicidal Ideation." *Suicide and Life-Threatening Behavior* 39, no. 6 (December 2009): 639–47.

Harrell, Margaret C., and Nancy Berglass. "Losing the Battle: The Challenge of Military Suicide." Center for a New American Society. October 2011.

Harvard T. H. Chan School of Public Health. "Means Matter: Attempters' Long-term Survival." www.hsph.harvard.edu/means-matter/means -matter/survival.

———. "Means Matter: Firearm Access Is a Risk Factor for Suicide." Accessed 4 September 2019. https://www.hsph.harvard.edu/means -matter/means-matter.

Hayes, Lindsay M. *Avoiding Obstacles to Prevention*. National Center on Institutions and Alternatives. 2011.

———. *Checklist for the "Suicide-Resistant" Design of Correctional Facilities*. National Center on Institutions and Alternatives. 2011.

———. *Guide to Developing and Revising Suicide Prevention Protocols within Juvenile Facilities*. National Center on Institutions and Alternatives. 2011.

Herrel, R., J. Goldberg, W. R. True, et al. "Sexual Orientation and Suicidality: A Co-Twin Control Study in Adult Men." *Archives of General Psychiatry* 56, no. 10 (October 1999): 867–74.

Heyman, Miriam, Jeff Dill, and Robert Douglas. *Study: Police Officers and Firefighters Are More Likely to Die by Suicide than in the Line of Duty*. Ruderman White Paper on Mental Health and Suicide of First Responders. April 2018.

Hoge, C. W., C. A. Castro, S. C. Messer, et al. "Combat Duty in Iraq and Afghanistan, Mental Health Problems, and Barriers to Care." *New England Journal of Medicine* 351, no. 1 (July 2004): 13–22.

Hoyer, G., and E. Lund. "Suicide among Women Related to Number of Children in Marriage." *Archives of General Psychiatry* 50 (1993): 134–37.

Hutson, H. Range, Deirdre Anglin, John Yarborough, et al. "Suicide by Cop." *Annals of Emergency Medicine* 32, no. 6 (1998): 665–69.

Ilgen, Mark A., Amy S. B. Bohnert, Dara Ganoczy, et al. "Opioid Dose and Risk of Suicide." National Center for Biotechnology Information. 1 May 2017.

Ilgen, Mark, and Felicia Kleinberg. "The Link between Substance Abuse, Violence, and Suicide." *Psychiatric Times*, 21 January 2011.

Institute for Criminal Policy Research. "World Prison Brief: Highest to Lowest Prison Population Total." Accessed 30 May 2017. www .prisonstudies.org/highest-to-lowest/prison-population-total.

James, S. E., J. L. Herman, S. Rankin, et al. *The Report of the 2015 U.S. Transgender Survey*. National Center for Transgender Equality. 2016.

Johns Hopkins Bloomberg School of Public Health. "CDC Provisional Data: Gun Suicides Reach All-Time High in 2022, Gun Homicides Down Slightly from 2021." 27 July 2023.

Johns Hopkins University Gazette. "John Hopkins Team Identifies Genetic Link to Attempted Suicide." 23 May 2011.

Joiner, T. E., J. S. Brown, and L. R. Wingate. "The Psychology and Neurobiology of Suicidal Behavior." *Annual Review of Psychology* 56 (February 2005): 287–314.

Joiner, T. E., Jr., and D. M. Rudd. "Negative Attributional Style for Interpersonal Events and the Occurrence of Severe Interpersonal Disruptions as Predictors of Self-Reported Suicidal Ideation." *Suicide and Life-Threatening Behavior* 25, no. 2 (Summer 1995): 297–304.

Joiner, T. E., Jr., D. M. Rudd, and M. H. Rajab. "The Modified Scale for Suicidal Ideation." *Journal of Abnormal Psychology* 106, no. 2 (1997): 260–65.

Joiner, T. E., Jr., and K. A. Van Orden. "The Interpersonal-Psychological Theory of Suicidal Behavior Indicates Specific and Crucial Psychotherapeutic Targets." *Internal Journal of Cognitive Therapy* 1, no. 1 (2008): 80–89.

Juhnke, Gerald A., Paul F. Granello, and Maritza Lebron-Striker. "IS PATH WARM? A Suicide Assessment Mnemonic for Counselors." American Counseling Association, *Professional Counseling Digest*, 2007.

Kang, Han K., and Tim A. Bullman. "Risk of Suicide among US Veterans after Returning from the Iraq or Afghanistan War Zones." *JAMA* 300, no. 6 (2008): 652–53.

Kaplan, Mark S., Nathalie Huguet, Benson H. McFarland, and Jason T. Newsom. "Suicide among Male Veterans: A Prospective Population-Based Study." *Journal of Epidemiology and Community Health* 61, no. 7 (July 2007): 619–24.

Kasen, Stephanie, Patricia Cohen, and Henian Chen. "Developmental Course of Impulsivity and Capability from Age 10 to Age 25 as Related to Trajectory of Suicide Attempt in a Community Cohort." *Suicide and Life-Threatening Behavior* 41, no. 2 (April 2011): 180–92.

Kreitman, N. "The Coal Gas Story: United Kingdom Suicide Rates, 1960–71." *Journal of Preventative Medicine* 30, no. 2 (June 1976): 86–93.

Lassne, Deborah, and Christine Yanez. *Repetition and Power Imbalance in Bullying Victimization at School.* Data Point. US Department of Education NCES 2018-093. March 2018. https://nces.ed.gov/pubs2018 /2018093.pdf.

Lawrence, Ryan E., Maria A. Oquendo, and Barbara Stanley. "Religion and Suicide Risk: A Systematic Review." *Archives of Suicide Research* 20, no. 1 (2016): 1–21.

Layman, Deborah M., Jamie Kammer, Emily Leckman-Westin, et al. "The Relationship between Suicidal Behaviors and Zero Suicide Organizational Best Practices in Outpatient Mental Health Clinics." *Psychiatric Services* 72, no. 10 (October 2021): 1118–25.

Leenaars, Antoon A. "Lives and Deaths: Biographical Notes on Selections of the Works of Edwin S. Shneidman." *Suicide and Life-Threatening Behavior* 40, no. 5 (November 2010): 476–91.

Lester, David, and M. E. Merrell. "The Influence of Gun Control Laws on Suicidal Behavior." *American Journal of Psychiatry* 137 (1980): 121–22.

Lindqvist, P., A. Jonsson, A. Eriksson, A. Hedelin, and U. Bjornstig. "Are Suicides by Jumping Off Bridges Preventable? An Analysis of 50 Cases from Sweden." *Accident Analysis and Prevention* 36, no. 4 (2004): 691–94.

Lubin, Gad, Nomi Werbeloff, Demian Halperin, et al. "Decrease in Suicide Rates after a Change of Policy Reducing Access to Firearms in Adolescents: A Naturalistic Epidemiological Study." *Suicide and Life-Threatening Behavior* 40, no. 5 (October 2010): 421–24.

Mann, J. John, Alan Apter, Jose Bertolote, et al. "Suicide Prevention Strategies: A Systematic Review." *JAMA* 294, no. 16 (October 2005): 2064–74.

Marin County Coroner's Office and the Bridge Rail Foundation. *A Fifteen-Year Report: Golden Gate Bridge Suicide Demographics.* September 2009.

———. *A Ten-Year Report: Golden Gate Bridge Suicide Demographics.* 2007.

Matasubayashi, Tetsuya, Y. Sawada, and M. Ueda. "Does the Installation of Blue Lights on Train Platforms Prevent Suicide? A Before-and-after Observational Study from Japan." *Journal of Affective Disorders* 147, nos. 1–3 (May 2013): 385–88.

———. "Does the Installation of Blue Lights on Train Platforms Shift Suicide to Another Station? Evidence from Japan." *Journal of Affective Disorders* 169 (December 2014): 57–60.

McIntosh, Wendy LiKam Wa; Erica Spies, Deborah M. Stone, et al. "Suicide Rates by Occupational Group—17 States, 2012." Centers for Disease Control and Prevention, *Morbidity and Mortality Weekly Report,* 1 July 2016.

Meier, Diane E. "The Treatment of Patients with Unbearable Suffering—The Slippery Slope Is Real." *JAMA Internal Medicine* 181, no. 2 (2021): 160–61.

Miller, Matthew, D. Azrael, and David Hemenway. "Belief in the Inevitability of Suicide: Results from a National Survey." *Suicide and Life-Threatening Behavior* 36, no. 1 (February 2006): 1–11.

Miller, Matthew, Catherine Barber, Deborah Azrael, et al. "Suicide among US Veterans: A Prospective Study of 500,000 Middle-aged and Elderly Men." *American Journal of Epidemiology* 170, no. 4 (May 2009): 494–500.

Miller, Matthew, and Hemenway, David. "Guns and Suicide in the United States." *New England Journal of Medicine* 359, no. 10 (September 2008): 989–91.

———. "The Relationship between Firearms and Suicide: A Review of the Literature." *Aggression and Violent Behavior: A Review Journal* 4 (1999): 59–75.

National Center for Health Studies. "Provisional Data Shows U.S. Drug Overdose Deaths Top 100,000 in 2022." 18 May 2023.

National Center on Institutions and Alternatives. *National Study of Jail Suicide: 20 Years Later.* May 2010.

National Humanities Center. "Suicide among Slaves: A 'Very Last Resort.'" In "The Making of African American Identity, Vol. 1: 1500–1865." www .nationalhumanitiescenter.org/pds.

National Suicide Prevention Lifeline. *Final Report of the Attempt Survivor Advisory Summit Meeting and Individual Interviews.* 2007.

New York State Bridge Authority. *A Comprehensive Plan for Suicide Prevention: Briefing and Summary Report for Consideration by Transportation Agencies.* 2008.

Niederkrotenthaler, T. "Role of Media Reports in Completed and Prevented Suicide: Werther v. Papageno Effects." *British Journal of Psychiatry* 197, no. 3 (September 2010): 234–43.

Nock, M. K., and P. M. Marzuk. "Murder-Suicide: Phenomenology and Clinical Implications." In *Harvard Medical School Guide to Suicide*

Assessment and Intervention, ed. D. G. Jacobs, 188–209. San Francisco: Jossey-Bass, 1999.

O'Carroll, P. W., and M. M. Silverman. "Community Suicide Prevention: The Effectiveness of Bridge Barriers." *Suicide and Life-Threatening Behavior* 24, no. 1 (1994): 89–91.

Omer, Haim, and Avshalom C. Elitzur. "What Would You Say to the Person on the Roof? A Suicide Prevention Text." *Suicide and Life-Threatening Behavior* 31, no. 2 (Summer 2001): 129–39.

Oquendo, Maria A. "Suicide: A Silent Contributor to Opioid-Overdose Deaths." *New England Journal of Medicine* 378, no. 17 (April 2018): 1567–69.

Orbach, Israel. "How Would You Listen to the Person on the Roof? A Response to H. Omer and A. Elitzur." *Suicide and Life-Threatening Behavior* 31, no. 2 (Summer 2001): 140–43.

Owens, D., J. Horricks, and A. House. "Fatal and Non-fatal Repetition of Self-harm: Systematic Review," *British Journal of Psychiatry* 181 (2002): 193–99.

Pelletier, Andrew. "Preventing Suicide by Jumping: The Effect of a Bridge Safety Fence." *Injury Prevention* 13, no. 1 (2007): 57–59.

Pestian, John. "A Conversation with Edwin Shneidman." *Suicide and Life-Threatening Behavior* 40, no. 5 (November 2010): 516–23.

Pew Research Center. *Muslim Publics Share Concerns about Extremist Groups.* Survey Report. 10 September 2013.

Phillips, David. "The Influence of Suggestion on Suicide: Substantive and Theoretical Implications of the Werther Effect." *American Sociological Review* 39 (June 1974): 340–54.

Qin, P., and P. B. Mortensen. "The Impact of Parental Status on the Risk of Completed Suicide." *Archives of General Psychiatry* 60 (2003): 797–802.

Qin, Ping, and Merete Nordentoft. "Suicide Risk in Relation to Psychiatric Hospitalization: Evidence Based on Longitudinal Registers," *Archives of General Psychiatry* 62, no. 4 (April 2005): 427–32.

Ramchand, Rajeev, Lisa H. Jaycox, and Patricia Ebener. "Suicide Prevention Hotlines in California: Diversity in Services, Structure, and Organization and the Potential Challenges Ahead." Rand Corporation. 2016.

Ramesh, Taanvi. "Suicide in Prison: A New Study on Risk Factors in the Prison Environment." Penal Reform International. 13 June 2018.

Reger, Mark A., Ian H. Stanley, and Thomas E. Joiner. "Suicide Mortality and Coronavirus Disease 2019—A Perfect Storm?" *JAMA Psychiatry* 77, no. 11 (November 2020): 1093–94.

Reisch, T., and K. Michel. "Securing a Suicide Hot Spot: Effects of a Safety Net at the Bern Muenster Terrace." *Suicide and Life-Threatening Behavior* 35, no. 4 (August 2005): 460–67.

Reisch, T., U. Schuster, and K. Michel. "Suicide by Jumping and Accessibility of Bridges: Results from a National Survey in Switzerland." *Suicide and Life-Threatening Behavior* 37, no. 6 (2007): 681–87.

Rilkoff, Heather, Sarah Sanford, and Jan Fordham. *Interventions to Prevent Suicide from Bridges: An Evidence Review and Jurisdictional Scan.* Toronto Public Health. May 2018.

Rosen, David H. "Suicide Survivors: A Follow-up Study of Persons Who Survived Jumping from the Golden Gate and San Francisco–Oakland Bay Bridges." *Western Journal of Medicine* 122, no. 4 (April 1975): 289–94.

Satcher, David. "The Surgeon General's Call to Action to Prevent Suicide." U.S. Public Health Services. 1999. http://profiles.nlm.nih.gov/ps/access /NNBBBH.pdf.

Satel, Sally. "Stressed Out Vets: Believing the Worst about Post-Traumatic Stress Disorder." *Weekly Standard* (Washington, DC), 21 August 2006.

ScienceDaily. "Genetic Link to Suicidal Behavior Confirmed."7 October 2011. www.sciencedaily.com/releases/2011/10/111007113941.htm.

Seiden, Richard H. *Can a Physical Barrier Prevent Suicides on the Golden Gate Bridge?* University of California School of Public Health. 5 June 1973.

———. "Reverend Jones on Suicide." *Suicide and Life-Threatening Behavior* 9, no. 2 (Summer 1979): 116–19.

———. "Where Are They Now? A Follow-up Study of Suicide Attempters from the Golden Gate Bridge." *Suicide and Life-Threatening Behavior* 8, no. 4 (Winter 1978): 203–16.

Seiden, Richard H., and Mary Spence. "A Tale of Two Bridges: Comparative Suicide Incidence on the Golden Gate and San Francisco–Oakland Bridges." *Omega—Journal of Death and Dying* 14, no. 3 (May 1984).

Shepard, Donald S., Deborah Gurewich, Aung K. Lwin, et al. "Suicide and Suicidal Attempts in the United States: Costs and Policy Implications." *Suicide and Life-Threatening Behavior* 46, no. 3 (June 2016): 352–62.

Shioiri, Toshiki, Akiyoshi Nishimura, Kohei Akazawa, et al. "Incidence of Note-Leaving Remains Constant Despite Increasing Suicide Rates." *Psychiatry and Clinical Neurosciences* 59 (2005): 226–28.

Shneidman, E. S. "Perturbation and Lethality as Precursors of Suicide in a Gifted Group." *Suicide and Life-Threatening Behavior* 1, no. 1 (1971): 23–45.

_____. "The Psychological Pain Assessment Scale." *Suicide and Life-Threatening Behavior* 29 (1999): 287–93.

_____. "'Suicide' and 'Suicidology': A Brief Etymological Note." *Suicide and Life-Threatening Behavior* 1, no. 1 (1971): 260–64.

_____. "Suicide Notes Reconsidered." *Psychiatry* 36 (1973): 379–95.

Simon, T. R., A. C. Swann, K. E. Powell, et al. "Characteristics of Impulsive Suicide Attempts and Attempters." *Suicide and Life-Threatening Behavior* 32, no. 1, suppl. (2001): 49–59.

Sinyor, Mark, and Anthony J. Levitt. "Effect of a Barrier at Bloor Street Viaduct on Suicide Rates in Toronto: National Experiment." *BMJ* 341 (July 2010).

Slovak, K., and T. W. Brewer. "Suicide and Firearm Means Restriction: Can Training Make a Difference?" *Suicide and Life-Threatening Behavior* 40, no. 1 (2010): 63–73.

Stack, S. "Media Coverage as a Risk Factor in Suicide." *Journal of Epidemiology and Community Health*, 57, no. 4 (April 2003): 238–40.

Stapelberg, Nicolas J. C., Jerneja Sveticic, Ian Hughes, et al. "Efficacy of the Zero Suicide Framework in Reducing Recurrent Suicide Attempts: Cross-Sectional and Time-to-Recurrent-Event Analyses." *British Journal of Psychiatry* 219, no. 2 (August 2021): 427–36.

Steels, M. D. "Deliberate Self-Poisoning—Nottingham Forest Football Club and F.A. Defeat." *Irish Journal of Psychological Medicine* 11, no. 2 (1994): 76–78.

Stirman, Shannon Wiltsey, Gregory K. Brown, Masrjan Ghahramanlou-Holloway, et al. "Participation Bias among Suicidal Adults in a Randomized Control Trial." *Suicide and Life-Threatening Behavior* 41, no. 2 (April 2011): 203–9.

Stovall, Jeffrey, and Frank J. Domino. "Approaching the Suicidal Patient." *American Family Physician* 68, no. 9 (2003): 1814–19.

Substance Abuse and Mental Health Services Administration. "Utilization of Mental Health Services by Adults with Suicidal Thoughts and Behavior." National Survey on Drug Use and Health. 2011.

Suicide Prevention Resource Center. "Rate of Suicide by Race/Ethnicity, United States 2008–2017." Accessed 1 November 2019. www.sprc.org /racial-ethnicdisparities (site currently unavailable).

Tanielian, Terri, Lisa Jaycox, Terry L. Schell, et al. "Invisible Wounds: Mental Health and Cognitive Care Needs of America's Returning Veterans." RAND Corporation. 17 April 2008.

Ting, Sarah A., Ashley F. Sullivan, Edwin Boudreaux, et al. "Trends in US Emergency Department Visits for Attempted Suicide and Self-Inflicted Injury, 1993–2008." *General Hospital Psychiatry* 34, no. 5 (September 2012): 557–65.

Tomassini, C., K. Juel, N. V. Holm, et al. "Risk of Suicide in Twins: 51-Year Follow-up Study." *British Medical Journal* 327 (2003): 373–74.

Toomey, Russell B., Amy K. Syvertsen, and Maura Shramko. "Transgender Adolescent Suicide Behavior." *Pediatrics* 14, no. 2 (September 2018): e20174218.

Towl, Graham, and David Crighton. *Suicide in Prisons: Prisoners' Lives Matter.* Hook, UK: Waterside Press, 2017.

Trovato, F. "The Stanley Cup of Hockey and Suicide in Quebec, 1951–1992." *Social Forces* 77, no. 1 (September 1998): 105–26.

Turk, Elisabeth, and Michael Tsokos. "Pathological Features of Fatal Falls from Height." *American Journal of Forensic Medicine and Pathology* 25, no. 3 (September 2004): 194–99.

Uquendo, Maria A., and Nora D. Volkow. "Suicide: A Silent Contributor to Opioid-Overdose Deaths." *New England Journal of Medicine* 378 (2018): 1567–69.

Weigel, Randolph R. *Suicide: What Leads People to Kill Themselves?* University of Wyoming Pub. B-1182. October 2007.

Whitmer, Dayna Atkins, and David Lauren Woods. "Analysis of the Cost Effectiveness of a Suicide Barrier on the Golden Gate Bridge." *Crisis* 34, no. 2 (2013): 98–106.

Wilson, Laura C. "The Prevalence of Military Sexual Trauma: A Meta-Analysis." *Trauma, Violence & Abuse* 19, no. 5 (2016): 584–97.

Zouk, Hans, Michel Tousignant, Monique Sequin, et al. "Characterization of Impulsivity in Suicide Completers: Clinical, Behavioral, and Psychosocial Dimensions," *Journal of Affective Disorders* 92 (June 2006): 195–204.

News Articles and Other Sources

ABC Fox News Montana. "Spokane City Council and Fire Officials Pushing for Protective Barriers on Monroe St. Bridge." 9 August 2021.

Abrams, Abigail, and Melissa Chan. "Special Report: Guns in America." *Time*, 5 November 2018.

Adolpjus, Emell D. "NY Bridge Safety Summit Eyes Suicide Prevention Measures." *Engineering News-Record*, 12 October 2023.

Agresti, James D., and Reid K. Smith. "Gun Control Facts." Just Facts. 25 January 2017. www.justfacts.com/guncontrol.asp.

Alexander, Kurtis. "Suicide on the Rise with Temperatures, Researchers Find." *San Francisco Chronicle*, 24 July 2018.

Alonso-Zaldivar, Ricardo. "988 Suicide Phone Hotline Getting $282M to Ease July Launch." Associated Press, 20 December 2021.

Alter, Charlotte. "The Young and the Restless: Adults Have Failed to Stop School Shootings. Now It's the Kids' Turn to Try." *Time*, 2 April 2018.

American Foundation for Suicide Prevention. "AFSP's Position on Firearms and Suicide Prevention." Accessed 21 November 2017. www.afsp.org.

Andelman, David A. "How France Cut Its Per Capita Gun Ownership in Half." *CNN*, 26 February 2018.

Anderson, Scott. "The Urge to End It All." *New York Times Magazine*, 6 July 2008.

Antrim, Donald. "Everywhere and Nowhere: A Journey through Suicide." *New Yorker*, 18, 25 February 2019.

Archer, Dale. "White, Middle-Age Suicide in America Skyrockets." *Reading Between the (Head)Lines* (blog). *Psychology Today*, 6 May 2013. https:// www.psychologytoday.com/us/blog/reading-between-the-headlines /201305/white-middle-age-suicide-in-america-skyrockets.

Asimov, Nanette. "Stanford study: Homicide risk doubles with a handgun at home. The victims? Mostly women." *San Francisco Chronicle*, 5 April 2022. https://www.sfchronicle.com/bayarea/article/Stanford-study -Homicide-risk-doubles-with-a-17057145.php.

Associated Press. "For Some Troubled Visitors, National Parks Become Chosen Site to End Life." 29 June 2008.

———. "Maine 8th State to Legalize Procedure." 13 June 2019.

———. "National Parks Becoming Suicide Spots." 2 January 2009.

———. "Overdose Deaths Higher in Cities Than Rural Areas." 3 August 2019.

———. "Panel: Military Needs Gun Safety Measures to Limit Suicides." 24 February 2003.

———. "U.S. Navy Deploys More Chaplains for Suicide Prevention." 30 March 2023.

———. "U.S. Overdose Deaths Hit Record 93,000 in Pandemic Last Year." 14 July 2021.

Assuno, Muri. "42 Percent of LGBTQ Youth Considered Suicide in 2020." *San Francisco Chronicle*, 20 May 2021.

Augarten, Stan. "Subject: Suicide." *Columbia Journalism Review*, July/ August 1982.

Augusta Free Press. "Legislation Aimed at Reducing Suicide Attempts at Bridges Introduced in Congress." 5 February 2021.

Austin, Steve. "I Was a Pastor When I Nearly Died by Suicide." *USA Today*, 25 September 2019.

Baldor, Lolita C. "Military Suicides Drop as Leaders Push New Programs." Associated Press, 22 October 2022.

———. "Reported Sexual Assaults across U.S. Military Increase by 13%." Associated Press, 31 August 2022.

———. "This Is What It's Like to Be an Army Woman in Combat." Associated Press, 26 February 2014.

Baldor, Lolita C., and Robert Burns. "Military Suicides Up 20% amid Host of Challenges." Associated Press, 29 September 2020.

Ballard, Chris. "Love, Loss, and Survival." *Sports Illustrated*, 17 November 2014.

Barnhorst, Amy. "The Empty Promises of Suicide Prevention." *New York Times*, 26 April 2019.

Barrett, Scott. "Lawmakers Want Barriers Erected on Three Newport County Bridges to Deter Suicide Attempts." *Newport (RI) Daily News*, 8 March 2021.

Bartlett, Tom. "The Suicide Wave That Never Was." *Atlantic*, 21 April 2021.

Bastia, Arden. "Advocates Push for Suicide Prevention Barriers." *Warwick (RI) Beacon*, 4 March 2021.

Basu, Moni. "Why Suicide Rate among Veterans May Be More Than 22 a Day." *CNN*, 14 November 2013.

Baum, Dan. "The Price of Valor." *New Yorker*, 13 October 2004.

Bay Area News Group. "California Gun Laws Are Helping Lower the Suicide Rate." Editorial. *Mercury News*, 15 September 2019.

BBC News. "U.S. Suicide Rate Surges, Particularly among White People." 22 April 2016. https://www.bbc.com/news/world-us-canada-36116166.

Benedict, Helen. "Why Soldiers Rape: Culture of Misogyny, Illegal Occupation, Fuel Sexual Violence in Military." *In These Times*, 13 August 2008.

Bengal, Erick. "Officials Prioritize Curbing Astoria Bridge Suicides." *Chinook Observer*, 1 February 2022.

Benjamin, Mark. "Is the U.S. Army Losing Its War on Suicide?" *Time*, 13 April 2010.

Benson, Heidi. "Lethal Beauty: Saving a Life." *San Francisco Chronicle*, 5 November 2005.

Bergen, Peter. "America the Lethal." *CNN*, 2 October 2017.

Bernstein, Lenny. "Study Links Opioid Use, Mental Health." *Washington Post*, 27 June 2017.

Bishop, Greg. "The Search for Why." *Sports Illustrated*, 2 July 2018.

Blum, Andrew. "Suicide Watch." *New York Times*, 20 March 2005.

Bower, Amanda. "A Survivor Talks about His Leap." *Time*, 24 May 2006.

Bracho-Sanchez, Edith. "Number of Children Going to ER with Suicidal Thoughts, Attempts Double, Study Finds." *CNN*, 8 April 2019.

_____. "Suicide Rates in Girls Are Rising, Study Finds, Especially in Those Age 10 to 14." *CNN*, 20 May 2019.

Bracken, Kassie, John Branch, Ben Laffin, Rebecca Lieberman, and Joe Ward. [Interactive] "They Started Playing Football as Young as 6; They Died in Their Teens and Twenties with C.T.E." *New York Times*, 16 November 2023.

Branch, John. "What the Golden Gate Is (Finally) Doing About Suicides." *New York Times*, 5 November 2023.

Brenner, Keri. "Report: Marin County Suicide Rate Declines." *Marin Independent Journal*, 4 April 2021.

Breslau, Karen. "An Unblinking Look at Suicide." *Newsweek*, 20 October 2006.

Brock, Rita N. "Moral Injury: The Crucial Missing Piece in Understanding Soldier Suicides." *Huffington Post*, 23 July 2012.

Buckley, Madeline, and Paige Fry. "'You May Be Able to Save a Life': Deaths from Falls at Water Tower Place Raise Questions about Suicide Prevention." *Chicago Tribune*, 16 January 2020.

Buhrmaster, Scott. "Suicide by Cop: 15 Warning Signs That You Might Be Involved." *PoliceOne.Com News*, 6 April 2006. http://www.policeone.com/police-products/training/articles/84176-SuicideBy-Cop-15-warning-signs-that-you-might-be-involved/.

Bumiller, Elisabeth. "Active-Duty Soldiers Take Their Own Lives at Record Rate." *New York Times*, 19 January 2012.

Burns, Robert. "Air Force Suicides Spike to Highest Level in Three Decades." Associated Press, February 10, 2010.

_____. "Number of Military Suicides Up." Associated Press, 15 January 2013.

Cabanatuan, Michael. "Bay Bridge Suicides Feared." *San Francisco Chronicle*, 11 March 2006.

_____. "Bridge Directors Vote for Net to Deter Suicides." *San Francisco Chronicle*, 11 October 2008.

_____. "The Great Barrier Debate." *San Francisco Chronicle*, 9 July 2008.

Cahill, Brian. "Police Need Protection from the Risks of Suicide." *San Francisco Chronicle*, 22 May 2011.

Calabresi, Massimo. "The Price of Relief." *Time*, 15 June 2015.

Calder, Rich. "Barrier Proposed to Prevent Verrazzano Bridge Suicides." *New York Post*, 4 June 2019.

Campbell, Charlie. "She Lost Too Many Friends to Suicide. Now Her App is Saving Lives." *Time*, 9 October 2019.

Capps, Kriston. "Suicides Related to Foreclosure and Eviction Doubled during the Housing Crisis." City Lab. 20 February 2015.

Carey, Benedict. "Is the Pandemic Sparking Suicide?" *New York Times*, 19 May 2020.

Catholic Church. *Catechism of the Catholic Church: Revised in Accordance with the Official Latin Text Promulgated by Pope John Paul II*. 2nd ed. Vatican City: Vatican Press, 1997.

Centers for Disease Control and Prevention. "Suicide and Self-Inflicted Injury." National Center for Health Statistics. Accessed 30 October 2019. www.cdc.gov.

_____. "Suicide by Method." National Institute of Mental Health. Accessed 8 November 2019. www.nimh.hih.gov/health/statistics/suicide.

Christensen, Jen. "Living Near a Gun Shop or in a Rural Area Puts You at Higher Risk for Suicide, Study Finds." *CNN*, 6 September 2019.

_____. "Suicide Attempts by Black Teens Are Increasing, Study Says." *CNN*, 14 October 2019.

Cillizza, Chris. "8 Charts That Explain America's Gun Culture." *CNN*, 2 October 2017.

Clay, Rebecca A. "Preventing Suicide among Veterans." *SAMHSA News*, May/June 2006.

Coffey, C. Edward. "Pursuing Perfect Depression Care: A Model for Eliminating Suicide and Transforming Mental Healthcare." Henry Ford Health Services, PowerPoint presentation. Accessed 16 April 2013. http://www.rcpsych.ac.uk/pdf/Pursuing%20Perfect%20Depression%20Care-1-2.pdf.

Cohen, Sharon, and Nora Eckert. "Many U.S. Jails Failing to Stop Inmate Suicides." Associated Press, 19 June 2019.

Coleman, Penny. "120 War Vets Commit Suicide Each Week." 26 November 2007. www.alternet.org/story/68713/120_vers_commit_suicide_each_week.

Combs, Michael. "SRJC Student Survives Jump off Golden Gate Bridge and Is Thankful at Second Chance." *Oak Leaf* (Santa Rosa Junior College), 27 February 2023.

Cook, Gale. "A Marin Blueprint for a New Golden Gate Bridge Agency." *San Francisco Examiner and Chronicle*, 19 February 1978.

Curwen, Thomas. "His Work Is Still Full of Life." *Los Angeles Times*, 5 June 2004.

Czekalinski, Stephanie, and National Journal. "Black Women Key to Easing Military Suicides?" *Atlantic*, 12 June 2012.

Daley, John. "State, Doctors Get Welcome Allies in Suicide Prevention Fight: Gun Shops." Colorado Public Radio, 28 April 2016.

Dao, James. "Taking Calls from Veterans on the Brink." *New York Times*, 30 July 2010.

DeMarco, Donald. "Glamorize Death and Copycat Suicides Follow." *National Catholic Register*, 6 July 2015.

Department of Veterans Affairs. "VA Suicide Data Update," January 2014.

Deprez, Esmé E. "Smoke 'Em Out." *Bloomberg Businessweek*, 9 October 2017.

Dicke, William. "Edwin Shneidman, Authority on Suicide, Dies at 91." *New York Times*, 21 May 2009.

Dixon-Mueller Ruth. "Last Will." *California*, Summer 2021.

Dokoupil, Tony. "Moral Injury." *Newsweek*, 10 December 2012.

Donaldson, James. "Suicide Bridge Reduces Impulse to Jump.," *ABC News*, 10 September 2012.

Dotinga, Randy. "One Year In, 'Bird Spikes' Haven't Stopped Coronado Bridge Suicides." *Voice of San Diego*, 21 April 2020.

Dubner, Stephen. "The Suicide Paradox." *Freakonomics*, podcast, 21 June 2011. https://freakonomics.com/podcast/the-suicide-paradox/.

Ducharme, Jamie. "Almost a Third of High-School Girls Considered Suicide in 2021." *Time*, 1 May 2023.

———. "A Disturbing Trend on the Rise." *Time*, 18 June 2018.

Dunkerly, Erin. "The Gun Lobby Is Hindering Suicide Prevention." *New York Times*, 26 December 2017.

Duster, Chandelis, and Barbara Starr. "Navy Confirms 3 Sailors Assigned to USS George H. W. Bush Died by Suicide." *CNN*, 24 September 2019.

Dwyer, Jim. "If Guns Do Not Kill, Tax the Bullets." *New York Times*, 9 August 2012.

East Bay Times. "Bay Area County's Suicide Prevention Efforts Are Working." Editorial. 12 July 2019.

Echeverria, Danielle. "Suicide Likelier for Women in Homes with Gun." *San Francisco Chronicle*, 2 May 2022.

Echeverria, Danielle, and Melissa Newcomb. "'What Am I Doing Wrong?' Stanford System Struggles." *San Francisco Chronicle*, 11 October 2022.

Economist. "Why Suicide Is Falling around the World, and How to Bring It Down More." 24 November 2018.

Education Development Center. "3 Things College Campuses Can Do to Prevent Suicide." Accessed 2 November 2022. www.edc.org/3-things -college-campuses-can-do-to-prevent-suicide.

Edwards, Haley Sweetland. "The Drug Cascade." *Time,* 3 July 2017.

_____. "The Horror That Won't Stop Happening." *Time,* 4 June 2018.

Egelko, Bob. "Judge Told VA Stalls on Care While 18 Veterans a Day Commit Suicide." *San Francisco Chronicle,* 22 April 2008.

Elassar, Alaa. "The Son of an Iraq War Veteran Designed an App to Stop His Dad's PTSD Nightmares." *CNN,* 13 December 2020.

Elliott, Philip, Haley Sweetland Edwards, and Charlotte Alter. "After the Massacre: Will the Deadliest Mass Shooting in Modern American History Change the Debate over Gun Rights?" *Time,* 16 October 2017.

Emanuel, Ezekiel J. "Four Myths about Doctor-Assisted Suicide." *New York Times,* 27 October 2012.

_____. "Whose Right to Die?" *Atlantic,* March 1997.

Erdman, Shelby Lin. "Drug Overdose Deaths Jump in 2019 to Nearly 71,000, a Record High, CDC Says." *CNN,* 15 July 2020.

Erdozain, Dominic. "What the Founding Fathers Would Say about Mass Shootings." *CNN,* 8 April 2021.

ESPN New Services. "Heather Anderson Diagnosed with CTE in 1st Case for Female Athlete." 4 July 2023.

Evans, Nate. "Their Battle Within." *Los Angeles Times,* 16 June 2013.

Everitt, Lauren, Andrew Theen, and Gulnaz Saiyed. "Efforts Lag to Improve Care for National Guard Troops." *Washington Post,* 14 February 2012.

Ewe, Koh. "Here's Why Malaysia and Other Countries Are Decriminalizing Suicide." *Time,* 28 June 2023.

Fagone, Jason, and Megan Cassidy. "Prisoner Suicides in State Climbing." *San Francisco Chronicle,* 28 December 2019.

_____. "Prisons Chief Admits 'Suicide Crisis' after State's Report." *San Francisco Chronicle,* 9 October 2019.

_____. "Prison Suicides Soaring Despite Calls for Reform." *San Francisco Chronicle,* 29 September 2019.

Falk, William. "Editor's Letter." *The Week,* 30 March 2018.

Filkins, Dexter. "Atonement." *New Yorker,* 29 October, 5 November 2012.

Fimrite, Peter. "The Great Barrier Debate." *San Francisco Chronicle,* 10 March 2005.

Finkel, David. "The Return." *New Yorker,* 9 September 2013.

Fitzpatrick, Edward. "Advocates Question Why Newport Pell Bridge Funding Did Not Include Suicide Barriers." *Boston Globe*, 1 November 2022.

Freedman, Samuel G. "Tending to Veterans' Afflictions of the Soul." *New York Times*, 11 January 2013.

Friend, Tad. "Jumpers." *New Yorker*, 13 October 2003.

_____. "A Net, at Last, for the Golden Gate Bridge?" *New Yorker*, 28 March 2014.

Frosch, Dan. "Fighting the Terror of Battles That Rage in Soldiers' Heads." *New York Times*, 13 May 2007.

Gelineau, Kristen. "Australian 'Angel' Saves Lives at Suicide Spot." Associated Press, 14 June 2010.

_____. "Neighbor Saves Scores of Lives at Suicide Spot." *San Francisco Chronicle*, 14 June 2010.

_____. "Opioid Addiction on Rise in Sad Echo of U.S. Crisis." Associated Press, 6 September 2019.

Gelles, Richard J. "Why Not Tax Bullets?" *American Interest*, 7 February 2016.

Gibbs, Nancy A., and Mark Thompson. "The War on Suicide?" *Time*, 23 July 2012.

Giffords Law Center to Prevent Gun Violence. "The Truth about Guns and Suicide." Accessed 3 September 2019. https://lawcenter.giffords.org.

_____. "Universal Background Checks." Accessed 26 January 2017. https://lawcenter.giffords.org.

_____. "Veterans and America's Gun Suicide Crisis." Accessed 3 September 2019. https://lawcenter.giffords.org.

Gilmour, Jared, and Joshua Tehee. "Why Toy Guns—but Not Real Guns—Are Banned on the Las Vegas Strip." McClatchy News Service, 3 October 2017.

Glantz, Aaron. "Suicides Highlight Failures of Veterans' Support System." *New York Times*, 24 March 2012.

Glionna, John M. "Bridge's Deadly Allure Lingers." *Los Angeles Times*, 5 June 2005.

_____. "Renewed Focus on a Bridge's Deadly Allure." *Los Angeles Times*, 31 July 2007.

_____. "Survivor Battles Golden Gate's Suicidal Lure." *Seattle Times*, 4 June 2005.

Glover, Scott. "He Sold an AR-15-Style Rifle to a Mass Shooter. Now He Wants Universal Background Checks." *CNN*, 7 October 2020.

Gold, Jessica, and Megan Ramsey. "It's Not about Linking Gun Violence and Mental Illness." *Time*, 19 August 2019.

Gold, Michael, and Tyler Pager. "Father of Sandy Hook Victim Found Dead in Apparent Suicide." *New York Times,* 26 March 2019.

Goodnough, Abby, Margot Sanger-Katz, and Josh Katz. "Drug Overdose Deaths Drop in US for First Time since 1990." *New York Times,* 18 July 2019.

Graff, Amy. "Champion of Golden Gate Bridge's Suicide Barrier Dies at 92." *San Francisco Chronicle,* 10 February 2021.

Green, Erica L. "Surge of Student Suicides Pushes Las Vegas Schools to Reopen." *New York Times,* 24 January 2021.

Greenhouse, Emily. "The Neglected Suicide Epidemic." *New Yorker,* 15 March 2014.

Gregory, Alice. "R U There?" *New Yorker,* 9 February 2015.

Gulliford, Andrew. "National Parks See Suicide Upticks Each Summer." *High Country News,* 20 August 2013.

Guthmann, Edward. "Lethal Beauty: The Allure." *San Francisco Chronicle,* 30 October 2005.

Hamlin, Jesse. "Lethal Beauty: Family Grief." *San Francisco Chronicle,* 31 October 2005.

Harding, Robert. "Rep. John Katko Proposes Federal Grants for Bridge safety Nets to Prevent Suicide." 14 September 2019. auburnpub.com.

Harris, Art. "A Hard Look." *San Francisco Examiner,* 10 August 1977.

———. "Public Prescriptions for Golden Gate's 'Epidemic.'" *San Francisco Examiner,* 16 March 1977.

———. "Stopping Suicides." *San Francisco Examiner,* 3 March 1977.

———. "Suicide: The View from the Bridge." *San Francisco Examiner,* 2 March 1977.

———. "Would a Barrier Stop Suicides?" *San Francisco Examiner,* 13 March 1977.

Harvey, Mike. "The Golden Gate to Heaven: Suicides Go On as Bridge Still Waits for Safety Net." *New York Times,* 7 November 2009.

Hassanein, Rokia. "New Study Reveals Shocking Rates of Attempted Suicide among Trans Adolescents." Human Rights Campaign. 12 September 2018.

Haubner, Andrew. "New California Bill Aims to Ban Tackle Football for Kids 12 and Under." *CBS Sacramento,* January 9, 2024.

Hayes, Christal. "Silence Can Be Deadly: 46 Officers Were Fatally Shot Last Year. More Than That—140—Committed Suicide." *USA Today,* 12 April 2018.

Healy, Melissa. "The Stronger a State's Gun Laws, the Lower Its Rate of Gun-Related Homicides and Suicides." *Los Angeles Times,* 5 March 2018.

Hefling, Kimberly. "Iraq War Vets' Suicide Rates Analyzed." Associated Press, 13 February 2008.

Ho, Patricia. "Analysis of Caltrain Death Patterns Begins Long-term Study of Railroad Suicides." *Stanford Daily*, 19 November 2010.

Ho, Vivian. "Golden Gate Bridge Suicides Hit Record High—46." *San Francisco Chronicle*, 26 February 2014.

Hogenboom, Melissa. "Many Animals Seem to Kill Themselves, but It Is Not Suicide." *BBC News*, 6 July 2016.

Hollyfield, Holly. "Suicides on the Rise amid Stay-at-Home Order, Bay Area Medical Professionals Say." *ABC-TV*, 21 May 2020. https://abc7news .com/suicide-covid-19-coronavirus-rates-during-pandemic-death-by /6201962/.

Holmes, Kristen. "Suicide Deterrent Construction on Coronado Bridge to Start in 4 Years." *CBS8*, 21 June 2023. https://www.cbs8.com/article/news/local /suicide-deterrent-construction-on-coronado-bridge/509-943dec44-7e65 -4482-9735-8a96730ae2af#:~:text=Construction%20to%20install%20 the%20suicide,for%20help%20addressing%20the%20issue.

Holsworth, Joseph. "Serving in Two Wars Didn't Kill Me, but the VA Might." *San Francisco Chronicle*, 7 November 2021.

Houston, Will. "Golden Gate Bridge Suicide Barrier Delays Add $23 Million to Cost." *Marin Independent Journal*, 8 August 2020.

————. "Golden Gate Bridge Suicide Barrier Work Continues during Pandemic." *Marin Independent Journal*, 9 April 2020.

Howard, Jacqueline. "Gun Deaths in US Reach Highest Level in Nearly 40 Years, CDC Data Reveal." *CNN*, 14 December 2018.

Humphreys, Keith. "Can a New $76 Million Net under the Golden Gate Bridge Really Prevent Suicides?" *Washington Post*, 3 September 2014.

Hyde, Pamela S. "Suicide: The Challenges and Opportunities behind the Public Health Problem." SAMHSA PowerPoint presentation, Tucson, AZ, 2 August 2011.

Jaffe, Greg. "VA Study Finds More Veterans Committing Suicide." *Washington Post*, 31 January 2013.

Jamieson, Patrick, Kathleen H. Jamieson, and Dan Romer. "Can Suicide Coverage Lead to Copycats?" *American Editor*, 14 June 2002.

Jelink, Pauline. "Suicides May Top Combat Deaths, Army Says." Associated Press, 6 February 2009.

Johnson, Carla K. "Sobering Report Shows Suicide Rates Rising across U.S." Associated Press, 8 June 2018.

Johnson, Karen. "Don't Celebrate Suicide: Educate." *Denver Post*, 16 August 2005.

Johnson, Lizzie. "Finding Kyle: In Search for Answers to 18-Year-Old's Suicide, His Family Found a Mission—Helping Other.," *San Francisco Chronicle*, 10 February 2009.

Jones, J. "Skyway Safeguards Don't Deter Jumpers." *St. Petersburg Times*, 6 October 2003.

Jones, Maggie. "How Do You Actually Help a Suicidal Teen?" *New York Times*, 17 May 2023.

Jordan, Elise. "Why I'm No Longer a Second Amendment Absolutist." *Time*, 16 April 2018.

Kaiman, Jonathan. "At Japan's Suicide Cliffs, He's Walked More than 600 People Back from the Edge." *Los Angeles Times*, 22 February 2018.

Kaufman, Ellie, and Paul LeBlanc. "519 U.S. Service Members Died by Suicide in 2021, Pentagon Say." *CNN*, 20 October 2022.

Keteyian, Armen. "Suicide Epidemic among Veterans." *CBS News*, 13 November 2007.

Khalil, Ashraf. "As Suicides Rise, U.S. Military Seeks to Address Mental Health." Associated Press, 10 October 2022.

King, John. "Lethal Beauty: The Engineering Challenge." *San Francisco Chronicle*, 4 November 2005.

Kirst, Sean. "Suicide-Prevention Counselor Says Barriers to Jumping Should Be Considered." *Syracuse (NY) Post-Standard*, 5 April 2002.

Klein, Joe. "Ten Years After: A National Disgrace." *Time*, 25 March, 2013.

Kluger, Jeffrey. "Robin's Pain: The Mystery of Suicide—and How to Prevent It." *Time*, 13 August 2104.

Koopman, John. "Lethal Beauty: No Easy Death." *San Francisco Chronicle*, 2 November 2005.

———. "Lethal Beauty: The Talkers." *San Francisco Chronicle*, 2 November 2005.

———. "No Easy Death: Suicide by Bridge Is Gruesome, and Death Is Almost Certain." *San Francisco Chronicle*, 2 November 2005.

Kounang, Nadia. "America's Doctors Call for Strongest Gun Control Measures to Date." *CNN*, 13 June 2018.

Kramer, Anna. "Anxiety, Depression Mount in Bay Area." *San Francisco Chronicle*, 19 August 2020.

Krauss, Clifford. "A Veil of Deterrence for a Bridge with a Dark Side." *New York Times*, 11 February 2003.

Krieger, Lisa M. "On Tracks Lives Are Lost but Also Saved." *San Jose Mercury News*, 6 September 2009.

———. "Preventing Suicides at the Tracks." *San Jose Mercury News*, 24 October 2009.

Kristof, Nicholas. "A Veteran's Death, the Nation's Shame." *New York Times*, 14 April 2012.

KTVU. "Suicide Documentary Angers Golden Gate Bridge Officials." 19 January 2005.

Kucher, Karen. "Experts: 'Suicide by Cop' Cases Are Hard to Prevent." *San Diego Union-Tribune*, 8 May 2017.

Langmaid, Virginia. "Overall, Suicide Rates Decreased in the US Last Year—But Not for Everyone." *CNN*, 3 November 2021.

Langreth, Robert, and Rebecca Ruiz. "The Forgotten Patients." *Forbes*, 13 September 2010.

Law, Tara. "New York City Police Officer Dies by Suicide—the 10th NYPD Suicide in 2019." *Time*, 16 October 2019.

Lee, B. J. "Death by Web Posts." *Newsweek*, 27 October 2008.

Lee, Jooyoung. "What We Can Learn from Canada on Gun Control." *CNN*, 24 April 2021.

Lehane, Jamie, and Sandra Oxx. "Peace of Mind: RI Bridges Need 'Lockboxes.'" *Newport (RI) Daily News*, 8 May 8, 2021.

Leinwand Leger, Donna. "OxyContin a Gateway to Heroin for Upper-Income Addicts." *USA Today*, 28 June 2013.

Levin, Aaron. "Clinic Visits Common before Service Members' Suicide." *Psychiatric News*, 6 April 2012.

Lezra, Billy. "A Stranger Asked Me to Take Her Photograph. It Saved My Life." *Washington Post*, 19 November 2023.

Los Angeles Times. "Fatal Overdoses Drop after Crackdown on Pill Mills." 3 July 2014.

Luscombe, Belinda. "Things Are Never What They Seem." *Time*, 25 June 2018.

Ly, Philip. "PM Vows to Boost Suicide Prevention Measures at The Gap." *SBS News*, 9 June 2016.

MacFarquhar, Larissa. "Last Call: A Buddhist Monk Confronts Japan's Suicide Culture." *New Yorker*, 24 June 2013.

Maddan, Heather. "Lethal Beauty: Nine Suicides." *San Francisco Chronicle*, 1 November 2005.

Mahoney, J. Michael. "If Suicide Barriers Are 'Ugly,' Suicides Are Uglier." *Marin Independent Journal*, 15 December 1996.

Marech, Rona. "Armed with Kind Words and a Helping Hand, Golden Gate Bridge Patrol Watches for Hints of Despair amid the Crowd." *San Francisco Chronicle*, 13 March 2005.

Marin Independent Journal. "Two Jump off Golden Gate Bridge." 2 June 1996.

Marquardt, Alex, and Ellie Kaufman. "Suicide Rate among Active-Duty Service Members Increased by 41% between 2015 and 2020." *CNN*, 30 September 2021.

Marrero, Tony. "Sunshine Skyway Bridge to Get Suicide Prevention Barrier." *Tampa Bay Times*, 9 January 2020.

Maugh, Thomas H., II. "Suicides and a Bad Economy Go Hand in Hand." *Los Angeles Times*, 14 April 2011.

Maynard, Roger. "Australia Mourns 'Angel of the Gap' Don Ritchie, the Man Who Talked 160 Out of Suicide." *Independent* (London), 16 May 2012.

McKinley, Jesse. "Golden Gate Managers Vote to Build Suicide Net." *New York Times*, 11 October, 2008.

McPhillips, Deidre. "U.S. Suicide Rates Rose in 2021, Reversing Two Years of Decline." *CNN*, 30 September 2022.

_____. "With Gun Suicides at Record Levels in the U.S., Rates Differ Markedly by State Polices on Gun Safety, New Report Shows." *CNN*, 29 September 2023.

McQueen, Shannon. "Twenty Years after That Day at Columbine High School, I'm Still Asking: Am I Safe?" *CNN*, 19 April 2019.

Moakley, Paul. "Eight Questions." *Time*, 17 September 2018.

Morales, Mark, and Steve Almasy. "An NYPD Officer Has Died by Suicide. It's the 7th Such Death This Year." *CNN*, 28 July 2019.

Moran, Mark. "Suicide Barrier Sought for Golden Gate Bridge." *Psychiatric News*, 1 April 2005.

Morgan, Kate. "The Acute Suicide Crisis Among Veterinarians: You're Always Going to Be Failing Somebody." *BBC*, 10 October 2023.

Morgan, Sarah Blake. "As Suicides Rise, Army Brass Reassessing Outreach." Associated Press, 28 September 2020.

Moriki, Darin. "Exhibit Seeks to Stop Suicide." *East Bay Times*, 13 November 2016.

Morris, Pamela. "I Don't Want Another Family to Lose a Child the Way We Did." *New York Times*, 25 March 2021.

Moyer, Melinda Wenner. "Journey to Gun Land." *Scientific American*, Winter 2017–18.

_____. "'A Poison in the System': The Epidemic of Military Sexual Assault." *New York Times*, 3 August 2021.

Mullen, George, Bill Walton, and Jack McGrory, "Opinion: An Inexpensive Barbwire Barrier Could Stop the Coronado Bridge Suicides." *Times of San Diego*, 4 October 2023.

National Center for Health Statistics. "U.S. Overdose Deaths in 2021 Increased Half as Much as in 2020—but Are Still Up 15%." Press release. 11 May 2022. https://www.cdc.gov/nchs/pressroom/nchs_press_releases /2022/202205.htm

National Institutes of Health. "Advancing Maryland's Statewide Suicide Data Warehouse to Improve Individual and Population-Level Mortality Prediction and Prevention." https://grantome.com/grant/NIH.

Nauert, Rick. "Majority of Suicides Occur after Midnight." Psych Central. 8 August 2018.

Nevius, C. W. "Taking a Little Time to Listen Could Save a Life." *San Francisco Chronicle*, 20 August 2018.

New.com.au. "Train Suicides Spike after Rain in Japan." 27 September 2013.

News21 Staff. "Back Home: Nearly 1 in Every 5 Suicides Is a Veteran." *Denver Post*, 28 August 2013.

————. "Back Home: VA System Ill-Prepared for Residual Effects of War." *Denver Post*, 25 August 2013.

————. "Back Home: Women Warriors Face Daunting Challenges in Civilian Life." *Denver Post*, 29 August 2013.

New York Times. "Inside a Killer Drug Epidemic: A Look at America's Opioid Crisis." 6 January 2017.

Norrie, Justin. "New Fence at The Gap 'Just Not High Enough.'" *Sydney Morning Herald*, 26 June 2011.

Nowinski, Chris. "Troubling Trend." *Sports Illustrated*, 16 July 2018.

Nutt, Amy Ellis. "Suicide Rates Rose Sharply in US, Report Shows." *Washington Post*, 8 June 2018.

O'Donnell, Dorothy. "Catch Me If I Fall." KQED. 22 April 2014. https://www .kqed.org/perspectives/201404220735/catch-me-if-i-fall.

Ola, Mary Jo. "Hoan Bridge New Safety Measure Seen as Potentially Life-Saving." *WTMJ-TV Milwaukee*, 2 November 2023.

Olson, Robert. "'Jumping' and Suicide Prevention." Centre for Suicide Prevention. Accessed 7 November 2018. www.suicideinfo.ca.

O'Neill, Marnie. "Dark History of Beautiful Spots Where Hundreds Have Died." 16 June 2018. https://www.news.com.au/travel/travel-updates /incidents/dark-history-of-beauty-spot-where-hundreds-have-died/news -story/27720b63cf174316ed3d479f8ca25bf0.

Onyanga-Omara, Jane. "Gun Violence Rare in U.K. Compared to U.S." *USA Today*, 4 October 2017.

Oprah Magazine. "Back to Life." January 2019.

———. "The Best Way to Talk about Suicide." January 2019.

———. "The Connection Cure." January 2019.

Park, Alice. "Suicide Rates Rose in 2021 after a Pandemic-Era Drop." *Time*, 13 April 2023.

Paterniti, Michael. "The Suicide Catcher." *GQ*, May 2010.

Peck, Sarah C., and James Alan Fox. "To Reduce Risk of Mass Shootings, Help Prevent Suicides." *San Francisco Chronicle*, 30 May 2021.

Perry, Tony. "Grim Exit Lines Gathered into Book." *Los Angeles Times*, 8 September 2004.

Personal Defense World. "Small Arms Survey: The US Has More Guns than People." 20 June 2018.

Phillipps, Dave. "Issue of Firearms Hinders Veterans' Suicide Prevention." *New York Times*, 16 October 2020.

Pogash, Carol. "Suicides Mounting, Golden Gate Looks to Add a Safety Net." *New York Times*, 26 March 2014.

Prado, Mark. "Family Struggles with Death of Teen Son from Golden Gate Bridge." *Marin Independent Journal*, 23 November 2013.

Prior, Ryan. "One in Four Young People Are Reporting Suicidal Thoughts. Here's How to Help." *CNN*, 15 August 2020.

Psychiatric News. "'Zero Suicide' Practices at Mental Health Clinics Reduce Suicide among Patients, Study Finds." 19 March 2021.

Psychiatric Services. "2006 APA Gold Award: Pursuing Perfect Depression Care." 57, no. 10 (October 2006): 1524–26.

Quillin, Martha. "For NC Park Rangers, Confronting Suicide Is the Worst Part of the Job." *Charlotte Observer*, 15 November 2014.

Rabin, Roni Caryn. "Frequent Moves Increase Suicide Risk in Teens." *New York Times*, 1 June 2009.

Rafkin, Louise. "Survivor of Bridge Jump Advocates for Mental Health, Safety Barrier." *Bay Citizen*, 20 August 2012.

Rapaport, Lisa. "Suicide Rates Rising across U.S." Reuters, 13 September 2019.

Reuters. "Higher State Minimum Wage Tied to Lower Suicide Rates." 20 April 2019.

———. "Suicide Risks Shared across Borders." 1 February 2008.

Reyes, Emily Alpert. "Suicides in U.S. Hit Historic High in 2022, Driven by Increases among Older Adults. *Los Angeles Times*, 29 November 2023.

Richarz, Allan. "The Amazing Psychology of Japanese Train Stations." City Lab. 22 May 2018.

Ritter, John. "Suicides Tarnish the Golden Gate." *USA Today*, 31 January 2005.

Rivera, Eddie. "Temporary Suicide Prevention Fencing Cuts Fatalities at Colorado Street Bridge, but City Wants Acceptable Permanent Solution." *Pasadena News*, 26 September 2019.

Roach, Mary. "Don't Jump!" *Salon*, 9 February 2001.

Robertson, Michael. "Legends of the Fall." *San Francisco Focus*, January 1997.

Romo, Vanessa. "Truckers Line Up under Bridge to Save Man Threatening Suicide." *NPR*, 24 April 2018.

Rosenberg, Debra. "How One Town Got Hooked." *Newsweek*, 9 April 2001.

Rosin, Hanna. "The Silicon Valley Suicides." *Atlantic*, December 2016.

Ross, Carolyn C. "Suicide: One of Addiction's Hidden Risks." *Psychology Today*, 20 February 2014.

Rovner, Josh. "Solitary Lockup Is Widespread and Quite Dangerous." InsideSources.com. 28 May 2017.

SAMHSA News. "New National Strategy Paves Way for Reducing Suicide Deaths." 10 September 2012.

Samuels, David. "Let's Die Together." *Atlantic*, May 2007.

San Francisco Chronicle. "Neglect behind Prison Walls." Editorial. 30 May 2017.

_____. "The Worlds We Fail to See." 9 June 2018.

Santa Fe New Mexican. "Our View: Safety at the Gorge Bridge Has Been Neglected Too Long." 12 May 2021.

Sapatkin, Don. "Suicides Involving Opioids More than Doubled in 15 Years, Study Finds." *Philadelphia Inquirer*, 31 March 2017.

Satia, Priya. "Mass Shootings and the Arms Industry." *San Francisco Chronicle*, 15 November 2008.

Savacool, Julia. "Rising Suicide Rates among Female Veterans Show How Deep the Emotional Wounds Can Be." *Women's Health*, 25 May 2012.

Savage, Nico. "Big Solutions a Long Way Off in Train Deaths." Bay Area News Group. 28 September 2019.

Scannell, Kate. "Suicide—A Deadly Burden to Society." Bay Area News Group. 13 June 2010.

Schulman, Henry. "Healing Together." *San Francisco Chronicle*, 19 July 2020.

Scutti, Susan. "Suicide in US Rose 10% after Robin Williams' Death, Study Finds." *CNN*, 7 February 2018.

Seyrig, Maria. "Depression Care Program Eliminates Suicide." Henry Ford Health Services press release. Accessed 16 April 2013. http://www.henryford.com/body.cfm?id=46335&action=detail&ref=1104.

Shute, Nancy. "A Plan to Prevent Gun Suicides." *Scientific American*, Winter 2017–18.

Simon, Darran. "The Opioid Epidemic Is So Bad That Librarians Are Learning How to Treat Overdoses." *CNN*, 24 June 2017.

Simon, Robert I. "Just a Smile and a Hello on the Golden Gate Bridge." *American Journal of Psychiatry*, May 2007.

Soffen, Kim. "To Reduce Suicides, Look at Guns." *Washington Post*, 13 July 2016.

Solomon, Andrew. "Anthony Bourdain, Kate Spade, and the Preventable Tragedies of Suicide." *New Yorker*, 8 June 2018.

———. "The Mystifying Rise of Child Suicide." *New Yorker*, 11 April 2022.

Sorkin, Amy Davidson. "Guns and the City." *New Yorker*, 4 February 2019.

Spiegel, Alix. "Study: Female Vets Especially Vulnerable to Suicide." *NPR*, 4 December 2010. https://www.npr.org/2010/12/04/131797071/study-female-vets-especially-vulnerable-to-suicide.

Stanford Suicide Prevention Research Lab. *Novel Therapeutics for Suicide Prevention*. Video presented by Rebecca Bernert at a meeting of the American Psychiatric Association, San Francisco, May 2023. https:www.youtube.com/watch?v=zjmbRQODwPQ.

Steinhauer, Jennifer. "Military Sexual Assaults Increase." *New York Times*, 8 May 2013.

Stephens, Thomas. "Golden Gate Follows Bern's Lead with Suicide Nets." swissinfo.ch. 4 August 2014.

St. John, Paige. "California Suppressed Consultant's Report on Inmate Suicides." *Los Angeles Times*, 28 February 2013.

Stobbe, Mike. "Life Expectancy Drops as Suicide, Overdoses Rise," Associated Press, 30 November 2018.

———. "Suicides and Homicides among Young Americans Jumped Early in the Pandemic, Study Says." Associated Press, 14 June 2023.

———. "U.S. Suicides Hit an All-time High Last Year." Associated Press, 10 August 2023.

Storrs, Carina. "Saving Lives at 18 of the World's Suicide 'Hot Spots.'" *CNN*, 28 September 2015.

Stracqualursi, Veronica, and Amanda Watts. "Suicide Prevention Hotline: FCC Proposes New 3-Digit Number." *CNN*, 17 August 2019.

Stubbs, Roman. "After Concussions Ended Her Soccer Career, a Former Star Is Helping Girls Avoid a Similar Fate." *Washington Post*, 20 August 2019.

Swaak, Taylor. "How We Talk about Suicide after School Shootings Can Be Dangerous: Experts." *Newsweek*, 25 February 2018.

Swan, Rachel. "Golden Gate Bridge Barrier Offers Relief." *San Francisco Chronicle*, 17 May 2019.

Swanson, Barrett. "The Two Faces of Suicide." *New Yorker*, 16 January 2019.

Swofford, Anthony. "'We Pretend the Vets Don't Even Exist.'" *Newsweek*, 28 May 2012.

Talbot, Margaret. "Gun Shots." *New Yorker*, 12 March 2018.

Tanner, Lindsey. "Half of Fatalities Come from 6 Nations, Including U.S." Associated Press, 29 August 2018.

_____. "Rise in Suicide and Social Media Coincide." Associated Press, 15 November 2017.

_____. "Self-harm, Suicide Attempts Climb among Girls." Associated Press, 22 November 2017.

_____. "Teen Suicide Attempts Higher in Conservative Area." Associated Press, 18 April 2011.

Tareen, Sophia. "Pandemic, Racism Compound Worries about Black Suicide Rate." Associated Press, 11 July 2020.

Tatham, Chelsea, and Angelina Salcedo. "FDOT to Install Suicide Prevention Barrier on Sunshine Skyway Bridge." *10 Tampa Bay*, 9 January 2020.

Tavernise, Sabrina. "Suicides Account for Most U.S. Gun Deaths." *New York Times*, 14 February 2013.

Taylor, Anita Darcel. "By My Own Hand." *Bellevue Literary Review* 6, no. 2 (Fall 2006): 117–21.

Thompson, Mark. "Is the U.S. Army Losing Its War on Suicide?" *Time*, 13 April 2010.

Torre, Pablo S. "A Light in the Darkness." *Sports Illustrated*, 21 June 2010.

Torres, Stacy. "No, I'm Not 'Fine,' and There Are Millions Like Me." *San Francisco Chronicle*, 19 June 2022.

Tracey, Julia Park. "My Son Took His Own Life. Here's Why You Should Stop Saying 'Committed Suicide.'" *Huffington Post*, 1 March 2021.

Trevor Project. www.thetrevorproject.org.

Trumbull, Todd. "Lethal Beauty: The Allure." *San Francisco Chronicle*, 30 October 2005.

Tyson, Bernard J. "Using Big Data to Help Stop Suicides and Self-Harm." *Time*, January 2019.

Uquendo, Maria. "Opioid Use Disorders and Suicide: A Hidden Tragedy." Congressional briefing, 6 April 2017. National Institute on Drug Abuse. www.drugabuse.gov.

Vainshtein, Annie. "Plans in Motion to Build Model of Golden Gate Bridge Suicide Net." *San Francisco Chronicle*, 30 August 2022.

Vick, Karl. "The Golden Gate: A Bridge Too Deadly?" *Washington Post*, 3 March 2008.

Vitelli, Romeo. "Are We Facing a Post-COVID-19 Suicide Epidemic?" *Psychology Today*, 7 June 2020.

Wadman, Meredith. "The Gun Fighter." *Scientific American*, Winter 2017–18.

Wan, William. "Chesapeake Bay Bridge Suicide; Preventing Jumps after Man Tries Twice." *Washington Post*, 7 September 2022.

Wang, Selina, Rebecca Wright, and Yoko Wakatsuki. "In Japan, More People Died from Suicide Last Month than from Covid in All of 2020." *CNN*, 29 November 2020.

Washington State Department of Health. "Suicide Prevention Training for Health Professionals: State of Washington Health Profession Mandatory Suicide Prevention Training." Accessed 18 October 2019. www.doh.wa.gov.

The Week. "Armed and Dangerous." 27 October 2017.

_____. "A Gunman's Deadly Rampage in a Texas Church." 17 November 2017.

_____. "Guns: Will Any New Laws Make a Difference?" 16 August 2019.

_____. "Netherlands: Should a Mentally Ill Teen Be Allowed to Die?" 21 June 2019.

_____. "Newtown, Conn., and Parkland, Fla. Horrors Persist." 5 April 2019.

_____. "Noted." 11 January 2019.

_____. "The Rise of White Supremacist Terrorism." 29 March 2019.

_____. "The Spread of Assisted Suicide." 20 March 2020.

_____. "Suicide: America's Hidden Epidemic." 22 June 2018.

_____. "Teen Suicides on the Rise." 1 June 2018.

_____. "Video Games and Violence." 20 September 2019.

Weiss, Haley. "Scientists Are Better Understanding the Link between Traumatic Brain Injury and Suicide." *Time*, 1 August 2023.

Weiss, Mike. "Lethal Beauty: A Survivor's Story." *San Francisco Chronicle*, 1 November 2005.

West, Emily R. "Design Work to Start for Barriers on the Natchez Trace Bridge." *Nashville Tennessean*, 6 January 2020.

Whiting, Sam. "Bernard Mayes—Former Priest, Radio Correspondent Started First Suicide Hotline in Nation in S.F." *San Francisco Chronicle*, 29 October 2014.

———. "A Resource of Hope for Mental Healing." *San Francisco Chronicle*, 15 May 2021.

Whyno, Stephen. "Weight Watching, Injury Dangers, Caustic Feedback Add to Mental Health Woes for Horseracing Jockeys." Associated Press, 23 May 2023.

Wiener, Jocelyn. "Treatment for Mental Illness Differs Drastically by County." Bay Area News Group. 8 July 2019.

Wild, Whitney, Paul LeBlanc, and Rashard Rose. "2 More Police Officers Who Responded to Capitol Insurrection Have Died by Suicide." *CNN*, August 3, 2021.

Williams, David. "Wisconsin Farmers Turned Their Corn Maze into an 11-Acre Billboard for a Suicide Helpline." *CNN*, 2 August 2019.

Williams, Timothy P. "Suicides Outpacing War Deaths for Troops." *New York Times*, 8 June 2012.

Wills, Garry. "Spiking the Gun Myth." *New York Times*, 10 September 2000.

Wong, Ashley, and Michael Gold. "Fourth Suicide at the Vessel Leads to Calls for Higher Barriers." *New York Times*, 29 July 2021.

Wong, Kristina. "New Report: Military Losing the Battle against Suicide." *ABC News*, 2 November 2011.

Worthington, Leah. "Slippery Slopes and Other Concerns." *California*, Summer 2021.

Yang, Jeff. "The Second Amendment Solution to Gun Violence." *CNN*, 7 August 2019.

Yuasa, Shino. "With Suicides a Concern, Japan Tries Mood Lights." Associated Press, 5 November 2009.

Zinko, Carolyne. "Lethal Beauty: An Inside Look at Who Jumps." *San Francisco Chronicle*, 31 July 2007.

———. "Lethal Beauty: The Advocate." *San Francisco Chronicle*, 3 November 2005.

———. "Lethal Beauty: The Barrier Debate." *San Francisco Chronicle*, 3 November 2005.

———. "Lethal Beauty: The Bureaucracy Barrier." *San Francisco Chronicle*, 3 November 2005.

———. "Lethal Beauty: The Toronto Example." *San Francisco Chronicle*, 3 November 2005.

Zito, Kelly. "Shoes Represent Bridge Jumpers." *San Francisco Chronicle*, 28 September 2008.

Zoellner, Tom. "Gun Industry's Takeover Silences Group's Suicide Prevention Message." *San Francisco Chronicle*, 17 November 2017.

Zoroya, Gregg. "Army Suicides Rise as Time Spent in Combat Increases." *USA Today*, 12 January 2009.

_____. "Female Soldiers' Suicide Rate Triples When at War." *USA Today*, 18 March 2011.

_____. "Repeated Deployments Weigh Heavily on U.S. Troops." *USA Today*, 13 January 2010.

Index

About the Author

JOHN BATESON was executive director of a nationally certified crisis-intervention and suicide-prevention center in the San Francisco Bay Area for sixteen years. He also has been executive director of three university-run counseling centers and deputy director of a multicounty social-service agency. He served on the steering committee of the National Suicide Prevention Lifeline (now known as 988 Suicide and Crisis Lifeline) and was appointed to a blue-ribbon committee that created the *California Strategic Plan on Suicide Prevention*. His first book, *Building Hope*, describes the challenges and rewards of operating a busy, twenty-four-hour call center. His next book, *The Final Leap*, is about suicides from the Golden Gate Bridge. It was followed by *The Last and Greatest Battle*, a history of military suicides from the Civil War to the present. *The Education of a Coroner*, his last book prior to this one, has been translated into multiple languages.

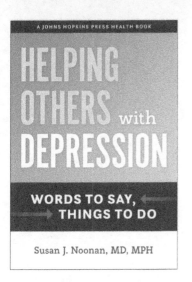
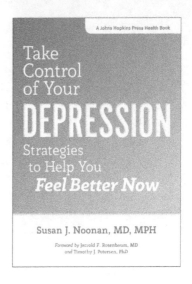
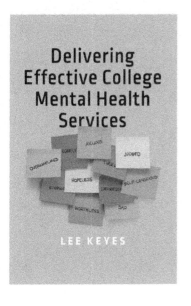
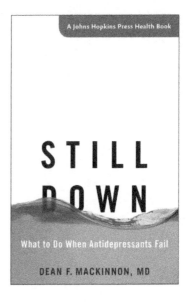